T0361894

Case Study Methodology for Nursing

This innovative text introduces and illustrates case study methodology for nursing research by exploring how it can be used to uncover the varied and complex life experiences of persons with chronic illness and post-traumatic stress conditions.

Nursing practice demands care and compassion, but often nurses do not have the tools to examine their clients' health and wellness experiences. This book presents an approach to finding shared solutions for common health problems from a nursing perspective. It provides readers with the tools to develop their own case study approach and the skills to translate their findings into innovative ways to influence nursing care for people across their health/illness trajectories. Rather than a prescriptive approach to care, it highlights the necessity of understanding what people are feeling, thinking, and doing to enhance health and improve quality of life.

This book is an essential read for nursing and qualitative health researchers. It is also an important companion for clinicians and academics concerned with caring for people with chronic illness and post-traumatic stress conditions.

Donna M. Zucker is a recognized expert in behavioral treatment for stress in incarcerated persons both in the United States and abroad, particularly those with substance-use disorder. She has developed several stress-reduction labyrinths for students, faculty, and homeless and incarcerated persons, to enhance health and healing.

Case Study Methodology for Nursing

Exploring the Lived Experience
of those with Chronic Health Problems

Edited by Donna M. Zucker

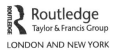
Routledge
Taylor & Francis Group

LONDON AND NEW YORK

First published 2024
by Routledge
4 Park Square, Milton Park, Abingdon, Oxon OX14 4RN

and by Routledge
605 Third Avenue, New York, NY 10158

Routledge is an imprint of the Taylor & Francis Group, an informa business

© 2024 selection and editorial matter, Donna M. Zucker;
individual chapters, the contributors

The right of Donna M. Zucker to be identified as the author of the editorial
material, and of the authors for their individual chapters, has been asserted in
accordance with sections 77 and 78 of the Copyright, Designs and Patents Act
1988.

British Library Cataloguing-in-Publication Data
A catalogue record for this book is available from the British Library

ISBN: 978-1-032-56407-4 (hbk)
ISBN: 978-1-032-56402-9 (pbk)
ISBN: 978-1-003-43535-8 (ebk)

DOI: 10.4324/9781003435358

Typeset in Times New Roman
by Apex CoVantage, LLC

Contents

Preface   *vi*
Contributor bios   *vii*

1 **Introduction**   1
   DONNA M. ZUCKER

2 **Meaning: Philosophy and theory**   5
   DONNA M. ZUCKER

3 **Case study methodology**   26
   DONNA M. ZUCKER, PATRICIA BRUCKENTHAL,
   AND MIKI PATTERSON

4 **Trajectories of health and illness**   36
   DONNA M. ZUCKER AND SHEILA PENNELL

5 **Self-care management**   41
   DONNA M. ZUCKER, ANNETTE MARUCA,
   SONYA LACHANCE, AND KIMBERLY DION

6 **Stigmatization**   50
   DONNA M. ZUCKER

7 **Application to clinical problem solving**   55
   DONNA M. ZUCKER, ANNETTE MARUCA,
   SONYA LACHANCE, AND KIMBERLY DION

8 **Current and future nursing directions**   60
   DONNA M. ZUCKER

Preface

This book emerged from my work with doctoral nursing students, whose own work in case study methods has informed my own. Across 20 years the compilation of case studies has highlighted the emerging need for this research, particularly in populations with chronic health problems who are marginalized from the mainstream healthcare system. Our hope is that the readers will come away with a sense of possibilities for their nursing practice. I want to acknowledge my faculty peers, former students, and my family.

Contributor bios

Dr. Patricia Bruckenthal is a nationally and internationally recognized nurse scientist, educator, and clinician. Dr. Bruckenthal has devoted her career to improving the assessment and management of people with chronic pain, improving care of older adults, and behavioral health integration.

Dr. Kimberly Dion is Clinical Professor at the University of Massachusetts Amherst. She is a harm reductionist and certified intranasal naloxone trainer for Massachusetts. Her broad and sustained impact is focused on decreasing substance-use disorder stigma, opioid overdoses, and infusing harm reduction education into academic and community programs.

Dr. Sonya Lachance is Online Maine School of Nursing Assistant Professor. She is multidisciplinary with 20+ years of experience as a technology leader. She is also board-certified in family health. Her research focuses on the use of technology in healthcare and substance use.

Dr. Annette Maruca is Associate Dean of Academic Affairs and Clinical Professor in the School of Nursing. She is board-certified in psychiatric mental health nursing and nursing education with extensive clinical and academic experience. Her scholarship is focused on behavioral health, corrections, and education.

Dr. Miki Patterson is a past president of the National Association of Orthopedic Nurses, recipient of an NIH grant, and former Associate Professor at University of Massachusetts Lowell in Nursing. Currently she is at 3M Hospital Information Systems Division developing Ambulatory Potentially Preventable Complications methodology software.

Dr. Sheila Pennell is Clinical Assistant Professor at the Elaine Marieb College of Nursing, University of Massachusetts Amherst. Dr. Pennell is an expert geriatric and hospice nurse and nurse educator engaged in teaching undergraduate nurses and supporting student and campus public health.

Dr. Donna M. Zucker is a recognized expert in behavioral treatment for stress in incarcerated persons both in the US and abroad, particularly those with substance use disorder. She has developed several stress reduction labyrinths for students, faculty, homeless and incarcerated persons, to enhance their health and healing.

1 Introduction

Donna M. Zucker

Definition

An accurate definition of case study methodology has significance for researchers. Unfortunately, it is a poorly defined concept in the literature and has been for decades. In a large integrative review of the use of case study methodology in nursing (de Andrade et al., 2017) authors found that 92% of the articles that met inclusion criteria used the term case study inappropriately as they did not adhere to case study methodology. The confusion may be due to the varied uses of the phrases such as "case report," "case study," or "case review."

According to D.B. Bromley (personal communication, May 6, 2001), the terms "case study," "case review," and "case report" are used loosely in the scientific and professional literature. The key features of a "case study" are its scientific credentials and its evidence base for professional applications. A "case review" might emphasize a critical reappraisal of a case. A "case report" might refer to a summary of a case or to the document reporting a case. Knowing the disciplinary context and meaning of these terms is important to convey to the reader.

In healthcare all these terms are used in various contexts. A "case report" in medical practice and advanced practice nursing is often synonymous with "case study" and may refer to the short beginning vignette of a person's bio-physiological signs and symptoms. It is disease specific and often reveals an unusual presentation and a unique trajectory. As the case study unfolds, additional signs and lab results create a clinical picture, potential diagnosis, and treatment. "Case study research" is often used synonymously with "case study methods." In nursing, "case studies" have a practical meaning and function in that they can be immediately applied to the participant's diagnosis or treatment and are useful in educating medical and nursing students (De Chesney, 2016).

Colleagues in the United Kingdom analyzed instances in which case study methodology was most appropriately used, employing a systematic, meta-narrative approach, reviewing various case study strategies (Paparini et al., 2021). Literature was examined for how each research approach was framed from pragmatic, pluralistic, historicity, contestation, reflexivity, and

DOI: 10.4324/9781003435358-1

peer-review perspectives, which helped identify four research traditions using case study methodology. This review included case studies that developed and tested complex interventions, that analyzed change in organizations, were appropriate for conducting realist evaluation and those that enabled naturalistic study of complex change. The authors noted that the first three approaches are informed by realist perspectives while the fourth is from an interpretivist orientation.

The aim of this book is to describe "case study the research method" as a useful methodology for nursing. If used accurately and consistently, it can provide an excellent description of the lived experiences of persons with chronic health conditions, not otherwise available through experimental and non-experimental methods alone. Case study strategies and research approaches discussed here will come from two of the most cited methodologists in the academic literature, Robert Stake and Robert Yin. In this book, the term "case study" connotes a research method.

Origins and uses of case research methodology

Nursing case study research approaches and strategies have been borrowed from the social sciences. Bromley (1990) described case study as a "systematic inquiry into an event or a set of related events that aims to describe and explain the phenomena (on) of interest" (p. 302). A key feature of a case study as a research method is the methodology itself. Yin (1994) has stated that the research design must have five components: the research question(s), its propositions, its unit(s) of analysis, a determination for how data are linked to the propositions, and criteria to interpret the findings. The method is mostly used prospectively, and data can emerge from documentation, archival records, interviews, direct observations, participant observations, and physical artifacts (Yin, 1994).

Across several editions of his books on case study research, Yin described a twofold definition that includes both the scope of the case study and the features of a case study. It is empirical, in-depth, and within a real-world context. It also may have features of other methodologies, relying on other sources of evidence (Yin, 2014). Cross-case analysis and pattern matching provide the researcher with "one of the most desirable analytic techniques, which compares the empirically based pattern with a predicted one" (p. 138). Yin concludes that a serious decision must be made to determine the best fit between case study research and other methods and then to follow systematic procedures, thus increasing the study's integrity.

Stake (1995) has proposed a similar model requiring a series of necessary steps for completing the case study method, including posing research questions, gathering data, data analysis, and interpretation. One difference is Stake's emphasis on a more naturalistic approach and the importance of philosophical underpinnings of the case method and of the description of contexts.

He states that cases can share unique and common qualities, and that case study method works well for people and programs and not so much for processes and events. Learning about a particular case is "an intrinsic interest in the case" (p. 3), thus the work is called an intrinsic case study, wherein the case is of highest importance. Alternatively, a case study could be undertaken to understand something other than the people or program of interest. The case study is then instrumental to accomplishing that and is called an instrumental case study. In instrumental cases, the issue(s) is of the highest importance. Studying more than one case is called a collective case study and some structures such as outlines of topical questions and issue questions are necessary. Stake also does not focus on quantitative case studies but rather the holistic, phenomenological, and biographical research methods.

Case study research in nursing

In a very targeted and focused review of the global nursing literature in using case study method, Steppe (2017) reviewed studies spanning 2013–2015 occurring across a broad range of settings: acute/inpatient care, long-term/elder care, community/outpatient care, mental health nursing, peripartum/prenatal care, professional development/workplace issues, and nursing education. The first authors were nurses. Themes that emerged were situations that included experiences of nurses in various settings: family members' experiences, studies evaluating workplace improvements, evaluation of an educational intervention in nursing education, interprofessional collegiality, and new nurse transition to practice. The findings were similar to those found in Anthony and Jack's (2009) integrative review of nursing studies utilizing case study method, who concluded that "there is evidence that case study research is being implemented in a rigorous manner and is entrenched in the nursing research lexicon as a well-accepted methodology" (p. 1179).

Most authors agree that central to meaningful case study research is the definition of what the case is. The researcher must be accurate, authoritative, and authentic, ensuring that the definition drives the methodology, and is concordant with the researcher's worldview. In that sense the case can be an individual, organization, community, or digital environment with limited or limitless boundaries. Chapter 2 focuses on the relationship between case study methodology and the underlying philosophy.

References

Anthony, S., & Jack, S. (2009). Qualitative case study methodology in nursing research: An integrative review. *Journal of Advanced Nursing*, *65*(6), 1171–1181. https://doi.org/10.1111/j.1365-2648.2009.04998.x

Bromley, D. B. (1990). Academic contributions to psychological counselling: I. A philosophy of science for the study of individual cases. *Counselling Psychology Quarterly*, *3*(3), 299307.

de Andrade, S. R., Ruoff, A. B., Piccoli, T., Schmitt, M. D., Ferreira, A., & Ammon Xavier, A. C. (2017). Case study as a nursing research method: An integrative review. *Texto & Contexto Enfermagem*, *26*(4), e5360016. https://doi.org/10.1590/0104-07072017005360016

De Chesney, M. (Ed.). (2016). *Nursing research using case studies: Qualitative designs and methods in nursing*. Springer Publishing.

Paparini, S., Papoutsi, C., Murdoch, J., Green, J., Petticrew, M., Greenhalgh, T., & Shaw, S. (2021). Evaluating complex interventions in context: Systematic, meta-narrative review of case study approaches. *BMC Medical Research Methodology*, *21*, 225. https://doi.org/10.1186/s12874-021-01418-3

Stake, R. (1995). *The art of case research*. Sage Publications.

Steppe, J. D. (2017). Chapter 2 – State of the art of qualitative case study methodology in nursing research. In M. De Chesnay (Ed.), *Nursing research using case studies: Qualitative designs and methods in nursing*. Springer Publishing.

Yin, R. K. (1994). *Case Study Research. Design and Methods* (1st ed.) Thousand Oaks, CA: Sage Publications, Inc.

Yin, R. K. (2014). *Case Study Research. Design and Methods* (5th ed.). Thousand Oaks, CA: Sage Publications, Inc.

2 Meaning

Philosophy and theory

Donna M. Zucker

Meaning and experience

For the clinician, it is essential to get at the underlying meaning a chronic health problem has for the patient. The combined efforts of medicine and psychology have revolutionized treatment for a wide range of chronic diseases, and can offer medications, invasive and non-invasive treatments, medical and surgical procedures, spirituality, psychotherapy, and self-care as key elements in the healing process. Yet, distinct and separate philosophies of care continue to dominate the treatment of several chronic health problems. Treatment compliance and practitioner perspectives lead the treatment process, but the descriptions of day-to-day events experienced by those who are living with chronic health problems is equally important to move the patient's experience along a wellness trajectory. Case study methodology is an excellent research strategy for getting at the meaning of the patient's experience.

Meaning model

Meaning refers to "the thing one intends to convey by an act or by language; the sense in which something (like a statement) is understood" Gove (1986, p. 1399). Meaning has many conceptualizations depending on one's philosophical framework. Burbank's (1992) model of meaning illustrates levels of meaning to capture these conceptualizations. The first level labeled meaning of signs and symbols represents a micro-perspective. At this very basic level, for example, persons can know the meaning of illness by viewing the face, walk, or talk of another. Level one may be considered a foundation or beginning of creating meaning.

The second level of meaning or midlevel of meaning, builds on the micro level and refers to the meaning placed on people, things, and events that occur across a person's life. It assumes that "a variety of things may be meaningful in varying degrees by different people" (Burbank, 1988, p. 13). Persons' responses to trauma, episodic illness, stigmatizing situations, and discrimination impact their meaning in life. This level will be discussed more fully in further chapters.

DOI: 10.4324/9781003435358-2

The third level is an abstract, macro level of meaning labeled "the meaning of life as a whole." Individuals may have no conscious awareness of this level of meaning, but rather function within a set of values and beliefs about life's meaning. Here a more existential or cosmic inquiry differs from "what is the meaning of my life?" which reflects one's need to have purpose in living. The latter may assist the patient to plan for the future given his current physical and psychological circumstances. Burbank equates "meaning of life" as a whole, as interrelated to the other two levels and is seen as one's worldview. She concludes that these levels of meaning encompass humankind's capacity to find importance in the experiences of living.

These levels represent the understandings of meaning from various philosophical perspectives, and these distinctions help to frame the subsequent discussion in terms of the "meaning in life" level for individuals with chronic illness. This level may operate based on an individual's beliefs and values and may include religiosity or spirituality. This umbrella level of meaning of life is not separate from but overarching the other two levels of meaning and informs one's worldview. In this conceptualization a human being can find the importance or meaning in the experiences of living. The next section will give a historical overview of various philosophical perspectives that inform meaning that coincide with each level: symbolic interaction, social constructionism, medical sociology, and existentialism. Each perspective has importance for nursing and case study research.

Symbolic interactionism

A variety of terms are used to refer to interactionism. Sometimes proponents are called "symbolic interactionists," "interactionists," "Chicago School," or "the Chicago tradition" (Fisher & Strauss, 1978). One's interactionist view can be microscopic focusing on the individual and his linkages to society, or more macroscopic focusing on fieldwork, and urban sociology. Often the term refers to the work of Herbert Blumer (1969), who coined it, or for George Herbert Mead (1934), who was the founding father and laid the basis for this perspective on society. The essential concepts to understanding this perspective come from his system of social psychology. Other Chicagoans have had a following similar to Mead (Everett C. Hughes, Robert E. Park, and W.I. Thomas). These traditions emerged between the years of 1910 and 1950. Meadian supporters have formed The Society for the Study of Symbolic Interactionism (Fisher & Strauss, 1978). Others outside this group are less narrow in their view.

Contemporary interactionists seem to fall into one of these two perspectives (Meadian or Park-Thomas), or a third group which has merged a little of both. In summary, various contemporary thinkers have borrowed portions of Mead's original work resulting in diverse theorizing, which has been thought to stem from controversies between the Iowa and Chicago Schools of interactionism. Turner (1991) discusses the areas of agreement and disagreement among these two schools outlining the views of Herbert Blumer and Manfred Kuhn, which are helpful in determining boundaries within which symbolic interactionists work. There are basic assumptions from which both stem. Human beings are symbol users and have the ability to read gestures and take roles as a framework for interaction. Emphasis is on the mind, self, and society (emphasizing the same capacities as Mead). Unifying these capacities allows for "interactions that form the basis of society" (p. 394). Certain concepts and ideas have been linked to each tradition: Thomas' "definition of the situation"; Park's process of conflict-accommodation-assimilation; Mead's concepts of "significant other," "role taking," and the "I-me" phases of the self. No matter which tradition one is speaking to, often the original works are cited as Mead's. His view of social change required him to develop a social psychology which focused on the progress of "civilization" as a whole.

This view functions as a kind of philosophic underpinning for the general interactionist perspective. A clear message of agreement from contemporary students of symbolic interactionism is the reference to the "active-actor," congruent with a changing paradigm: one that is anti-deterministic, and against functionalism and quantification in the social sciences. Students of these two traditions which are better known in the field of social psychology are Howard Becker (1966) (deviancy, occupations), Erving Goffman (1972) (social interactionism), and Anselm Strauss (1971) (social psychology, urban, occupations).

Origins of symbolic interactionism within sociology and psychology

Charon (1992) describes social science as a perspective which is made up of subperspectives. Three of these are sociology, psychology, and psychological social psychology. Sociology focuses on the social structure in its analysis. Berger and Luckman's description of the sociological perspective is "the human being as shaped and controlled by outside forces, by forces relating to social structure" (1967, p. 16). Its conceptual framework aims to isolate the important social regularities and to determine social cause (Sarbin & Kitsuse, 1994).

Psychologists have relied heavily on the controlled laboratory experiment and they have usually considered the human being wholly in the world of phenomena, moved by natural laws, created, and shaped. Although both sociological and psychological perspectives emphasize studying human behavior, psychologists focus on the individual organism and how it is shaped, whereas sociologists focus on social structure and how people are shaped by their positions in various social structures. In psychology cause for change is in what happens to or within the organism, whereas in sociology, cause for change is in the changes in the social structure, in changes in the person's position in that structure or in the person going from one social structure to another. Both views are deterministic.

The final perspective has two branches: psychological social psychology (PSP) and sociological social psychology (SSP). Psychological social psychology has its roots in Gestalt psychology which emphasizes the central importance of perception in human behavior. This discipline focuses on interpersonal influence, or how others influence our thoughts, feelings, and behaviors (Charon, 1992). The most important idea is that human beings are influenced by what goes on in the "social situation." Social psychology attempts to uncover the causes of human behavior by isolating forces in the social environment that create individual attitudes and behavior. The emphasis on the social and on the importance of the situation distinguishes social psychology from other perspectives in psychology, and the focus on the reaction of the person to the social tends to distinguish it from sociology.

Sociological social psychology has four foci. The first is on the ongoing interaction rather than on static concepts such as attitudes, acts, or perception. The second is an emphasis on how the individual changes in interaction over time. Third, there is a greater emphasis on research of real-life events. A fourth is a strong emphasis on socialization, or how the individual takes on the rules and views of society. Here SSP can be divided into two categories: the discipline of sociology in general and symbolic interactionism. The former can be divided into macrosociology referring to the study of large-scale organized life, and microsociology which is the study of small group life and socialization (Charon, 1992).

The second category is symbolic interactionism, which seeks to "explain human behavior in terms of symbols" (Spradley, 1979, p. 6). The four central ideas of symbolic interactionism are: the focus on the nature of social interaction; that human action results from interaction within the individual, that we act according to how we define the situation we are in; the focus is on the present, not the past; and finally this perspective describes the human being as more unpredictable and active in his or her world (Charon, 1992). Definition of the situation is seen as a middle range theory which developed out of the symbolic interactionism perspective.

W.I. Thomas, credited with coining the phrase, contributed that within the capabilities of the mind, persons engage in a process of examination and deliberation prior to any self-determined behavior. Definition of the situation may be an active emergent process of reality construction. It may also be conceived as an outcome, that is a point of view that results from defining the situation.

Social constructionism

Meaning is the product of everyday social interaction. Human beings are active agents processing information carried out in the context of cultural practices, purposes, and beliefs (Sarbin & Kitsuse, 1994). A constructionist perspective from sociological and psychological perspectives means that "constructionists focus on how ordinary members create and employ constructions in observing how others interact with those constructions and on interpreting and sometimes proposing alternate constructions" (p. ix). This philosophical perspective comes out of the influence of George H. Mead and others who pursued the theme of symbolic interaction. We accept many constructions of the basis of legitimate authority. For example, patients often seek out and accept a physician's opinion and help in getting symptom relief. They follow the "rules of the game" to whatever extent is necessary. To a certain degree, decisions about their illness trajectory are influenced by the doctor's knowledge. The doctor and the patient each define the patient's situation.

The sociological perspective of social constructionism suggests that "social objects are not given 'in the world' but constructed, negotiated, reformed, fashioned and organized by human beings in an effort to make sense of happenings in the world" (Sarbin & Kitsuse, 1994, p. 3). This is congruent with the philosophies of Schutz (1967) and Berger and Luckman (1967). The most widely practiced application of the constructionist perspective was generated by symbolic interactionists who have produced a substantial body of empirical research, primarily in the sociology of social problems (Becker, 1966; Schneider, 1985; Spector & Kitsuse, 1987). Social problems can be thought of as social ills or conditions which impinge on the social order. These may include poverty, violence, and racism. The description of social problems as both a subjective and objective activity continues to be discussed. Such works describe factors that impinge on how persons are naming what is happening to them. A hallmark of the social constructionist perspective is "that the essence of social problems lies in the activities of individuals or groups making assertions or grievances and claims with respect to some putative condition" (Hanrahan, 1995). From psychology, work in this area has come much more slowly.

Following criticisms of the reliance on lab experiments in which phenomena under investigation were de-contextualized, psychologists sought a framework to challenge the prevailing traditional ones. Hilbert (1984), one of the earliest psychologists to employ social constructionism in the health arena, describes a cognitive component to meaning making. Regarding chronic pain, he views reality construction as somewhat independent from culture due to pain's perceived location inside the individual, which cannot be verified from outside the body. In this sense, pain transcends a person's ability to experience it as a fact in the social sense, "that is as an item of knowledge" (p. 366).

Malone (1995) studied heavy users of emergency room services. She contended that two theoretical frameworks combine to support her notion that:

1) according to the social constructionist perspective problems are defined and created by our understandings of them, and 2) according to phenomenology, that such understandings are primarily experiential rather than cognitive.

(p. 470)

She concluded that social construction of social problems and articulation of solutions by varied key players in healthcare reform have divergent and often conflicting premises.

Meaning in life within medical sociology

The construction of health and illness is shaped by many elements often independent from biomedical phenomena. It links the varied manifestations of health and illness, biomedical data, medical practice, institutional structure, social policy, economics, epidemiology of disease and death, and individual experiences of health, illness, and medical care. Distinctions are made between disease and illness. Disease is a biomedical phenomenon strongly influenced by social forces (Brown, 1991) while illness reflects a more subjective phenomenon. People differ in their perception of illness and choose widely disparate ways of dealing with symptoms. Medical sociologists see much of illness itself as a social construction, that is, a phenomenon caused by human and institutional beliefs and actions, rather than solely by a value-neutral physiological process. If this is true, then standard medical treatment alone is not enough to impact or reverse chronic illness states. To illustrate this point, it has been shown that even small lifestyle changes can have a positive impact on health. Lifestyle medicine focuses on modifying unhealthy behaviors that contribute to declines in trajectories of health (Sadiq, 2023). These include activity, diet, stress, and other risk factors that contribute to poor health.

Morbidity and mortality of heart disease has been greatly altered by self-care measures to reduce cardiac risk factors. For example, the severity of distinct coronary lesions has been reduced following a regimen of vegetarian diet, yoga, and meditation (Ornish, 1990). While non-technological disease reversal is revolutionary, anecdotal evidence concludes that most individuals find following this strict self-care regimen as "too hard." Another study has demonstrated that factors such as social support affect illness behavior and the personal experience of illness, irrespective of health status (Kostis et al., 1992).

The boundaries of medical treatment must expand to include alternate treatments and explanations of illness care. Chronic illnesses are predominant health problems in our country, and non-compliance is a major problem for practitioners and patients. Instead of unwillingness to comply with doctors' recommendations, perhaps non-compliance is a deliberate form of avoidance of recommendations which impair personal or work life. Successful treatments for chronic illness must surely consider the patient's perspective.

According to Kleinman (1986), the experience of illness may "mean" in several senses. First, there is the overt meaning of the symptom, such as chest pain or shortness of breath. Such shared meanings are more or less standard in the culture. A second sense has to do with the cultural significance attributed to certain disorders in certain societies. Cultural meanings inform perception of bodily processes, behaviors, and habits. "These culturally marked disorders may bring meanings to individuals and the society at large" (Kleinman, p. 145). In the third sense, illness takes on peculiar meanings that differentiate our personal lives and interpersonal situations. "Illnesses may crystallize deep inner meanings (threat, punishment, loss) affecting one's sense of self and bind these to moral and religious aspects of suffering" (p. 146).

Because illness experience is an intimate part of social systems of meaning and rules for behavior, it is strongly influenced by culture; it is culturally constructed (Kleinman et al., 1978). Medical anthropology is focused on basic clinical questions to a greater degree than other social sciences. These researchers recognize clinical reality as culturally constructed and pluralistic, thus freeing them from an ethnocentric professional framework. Medicine must strive to link the doctor's explanatory model of disease with the patient's explanatory model of illness. "Systematic inattention to illness is in part responsible for patient non-compliance" (Kleinman et al., 1978, p. 252). "Illness reality" characterizes the process of the MD/patient encounter. This concept is seen as a " 'syndrome' of typical experiences, a set of words, experiences, and feelings which typically run together for members of a given society, a set of experiences associated through networks of meaning and social interaction" (Good & Good, 1982, p. 148).

For pragmatists, meaning is anchored in behavior. A pragmatic approach recognizes that phenomena in the mundane world have different meanings for different individuals. Here phenomena have meanings only insofar as they can be seen to link ongoing events for individuals. It is felt that when an individual is confronted with an isolated phenomenon in his immediate environment, he does three things. He isolates the phenomenon from other phenomena, he identifies the linkages the phenomena have with himself and with his present condition, and finally he predicts the consequences of the phenomena. Once isolated, all phenomena are potentially symbolic in their functioning in human affairs (Kleinman, 1986, pp. 225–226).

Existentialism

Among the three prominent schools of psychology (Freudian, Gestalt, and Existential), existential analysis is most suited to this discussion. There are links with this school to both symbolic interactionism and motivational theories, both having had a profound impact on the treatment of illness, both mental and physical. The gaps, however, which exist in this dualistic approach are addressed in logotherapy. Discovered by Victor Frankl (1963) in his writings following his internment in concentration camps during the Second World War, Frankl challenged the then conventions of psychotherapy to appreciate the existential aspects of the human being: the mind, body, and spirit (nooetic).

Frankl's perspective is conceptualized in a systematic way. Basic tenets are: (1) the freedom of will; (2) the will to meaning; (3) and the meaning of life. Freedom of will refers to the freedom human beings have to make choices regarding his activities, experiences, attitudes, and that his freedom permits him to modify himself – to transcend above the physical and psychological determinants of existence. Will to meaning refers to man's search for meaning as a primary force in his life, not an instinctual drive. Man's discovery of the meanings of his life is aided by certain values and traditions which are passed on from generation values and traditions which are passed on from generation to generation. This perspective seems most suited to address the ills of the post-war era, namely, boredom and apathy (Frankl, 1969). This "existential vacuum" refers to the patient's complaint of feelings of emptiness and meaninglessness. During the post-war period, many youths contemplating suicide viewed their lives in only one direction: the unemployed in finding work, the unmarried woman in finding a husband (Calabrese, 1974, p. 17). This meaninglessness is derived from two facts: man wishes to do what other people do (conformism) or he does what other people wish him to do (totalitarianism). Frankl believed that life holds meaning for each individual, and he retains this meaning literally to his last breath. The approach to assist patients is called "logotherapy" and the goal is not to show the patient what the meaning is, but to show him that "there is a meaning, and that life retains it; that it remains meaningful under any conditions" (Frankl, 1969, p. ix).

Unique to this school of psychology is the importance of the third dimension of humanness known as the spiritual (meant as the anthropological rather than the theological dimension). The uniquely human phenomena are located in this dimension. This can be illustrated in the following example. Despite the conditions of the concentration camps, Frankl saw the unexpected extent to which man was, and always remains, capable of resisting and braving the worst of conditions, by detaching oneself from those conditions. Man's capacity to do so is manifested through heroism and through humor. These two capacities are uniquely human ways of self-detachment, whereby man takes a stand toward his own somatic and psychic conditions. This leads to the spiritual dimension.

Human phenomena such as love, conscience, and self-transcendence are human capacities which have very unique meaning for each individual. Reductionist attempts at analysis disregard and ignore the humanness of these phenomena by making them into subhuman phenomena. Scientific reductionism exerts a similar influence on contemporary treatment of disease. For example, nurses strive to preserve the oneness of the human condition through health promotion and holistic nursing care, while medicine strives to diagnose and treat specific components of the human condition. Frankl (1969) contends if man is thought to be unity despite multiplicity, he is conceived in terms of bodily, mental, and spiritual strata. Practitioners must deal with man as though the somatic, psychic, and noetic modes of being cannot be separated from each other. This notion is congruent with a nursing philosophy.

Frankl's perspective contends that man is reaching to encounter the world, its beings, and others to encounter the meanings for fulfillment. This view contrasts with those motivational theories which are based on the homeo-stasis principal. The individual wants to create values and has a primary or native orientation in the direction of creating values. Man is pushed by drives but pulled by meaning, and this implies that it is always up to him to decide whether he wishes to fulfill the latter. Thus, meaning fulfillment always implies decision-making.

Frankl (1963) states, "the meaning of life differs from man to man, from day- to-day and hour to hour. What matters . . . is not the meaning of life in general but rather the specific meaning of a person's life at a given moment" (p. 171). Here Frankl makes no distinction between "meaning of life" and "meaning in life." "Meaning in life" can be discovered in three different ways: "by doing a deed, by experiencing a value, and by suffering" (p. 176). While the first way of finding meaning in life is self-explanatory, Frankl describes the second by elaborating on experiencing someone or love. Love is seen as spiritual and reciprocal. The third way of finding meaning in life is described as when one is confronted with an incurable disease. When all chances of life are erased, one is "given a last chance to actualize the highest value, to fulfill the deepest meaning, the meaning of suffering" (p. 178). We can choose the attitude we take toward suffering.

Conceptually, Fabry (1968) interpreted this to mean that all meaning is in the realm of three general areas: activities, personal experiences, and attitudes. Meaning can be provided through activities such as one's job, hobbies, and deeds done for the sake of others; participation is implied in these activities. The second area through which man can realize meaning is the area of experi-ences such as beauty, truth, or love; experiences provide man with meaning by receiving. Frankl asserts the deepest meaning can be found in attitudes. When a person encounters a difficult situation which cannot be changed, he can find meaning in facing it bravely, with dignity and by providing an example to oth-ers in a similar predicament. Man's attitudes, more so than his activities and experiences, allow him the chance to experience meaning through creative activity and personal experience. This leads to the notion of "ultimate mean-ing" in which beliefs exist on the highest possible plane. This idea has caused Frankl to be labeled with the accusation of "sneaking in religion by the back door" (Calabrese, 1974). These general areas have been interpreted as values. Frankl's later writings refer to "universal meanings" which are unique mean-ings for many individuals that correlate to societal norms. Frankl has equated these universal meanings with values (Burbank, 1988).

The fundamental weakness of logotherapy is the lack of any sound theoret-ical basis upon which it rests. It is best embraced as a therapeutic approach for persons lacking meaning in their lives. Calabrese (1974) critiqued the theory's basic assumptions by asserting that contemporary economic, political, and social developments have adversely affected man's sources of emotional well-being. He asserts that Frankl has made important observations and woven them into the basic tenets of logotherapy. For example, happiness or fulfill-ment is the by-product of the quest for meaningful goals, but anyone who seeks happiness as an end in itself will be unfulfilled. Calabrese claims that Frankl is not really able to explain why this is so, and since the central question of logotherapy revolves around the achieving of meaning and fulfillment, it is vital to see how these experiences came into being. Calabrese contends that the "existential vacuum" in modem western man is due to the stresses of industrial-technological culture, and the limitations imposed on man by his evolutionary design. Calabrese (1974) calls for a need to establish evolutionary biology as the fundamental basis of Frankl's perspective, which can direct its therapy. He cites the contributions of Levi-Strauss and Piaget as having emphasized the importance of basing the framework of social anthropology on man's biology.

Dubos (1970) maintained that man becomes gradually tolerant of worsening environmental conditions without having the insight that the expressions of this tolerance will emerge before long as debilitating ailments. Logotherapeutic techniques which help people find meaning in life utilize paradoxical intention, whereby patients are encouraged to face their fears; and dereflection, which is the purposeful avoidance of a painful behavior and a shift in focus to giving to others. This latter notion seems to be aligned with a strong Judeo-Christian ethic of spiritual transcendence from pain and suffering (Frankl, 1963).

Instruments have been developed to specify interventions for a variety of patient problems for whom logotherapy is recommended. The Values Awareness Technique (VAT) includes exercises which are designed to illuminate creative, experiential, and attitudinal classes of values. It is a paper-and-pencil technique for facilitating the process of revealing an individual's underlying value system (Hutzell, 1992). The Logo-test (an existential frustration measure developed by Lukas, 1991) has been used in combination with a variety of other psychological scales to determine experience-determined traits of frustration. This finding is interpreted as supporting the logotherapeutic conception of interaction between the "meaning in life" quality and personality dimensions (Balcar, 1995).

The logotherapeutic techniques called dereflection and paradoxical intention both rest on two essential qualities of human existence: man's capacity for self-transcendence and self-detachment. Logotherapeutic counseling techniques have been deemed particularly useful in family therapy (Lukas, 1991), with traumatized patients (Lantz, 1996), therapy with elders (Kimble et al., 1989; Brown & Romanchuk, 1994), with patients who have had substance use disorder (Wadsworth, 1992; Hutzell, 1992), and nursing home patients (Starck, 1992). According to Harper (1990), who has worked with patients undergoing "midlife crises," existential vacuum is synonymous with depression.

Joyce Travelbee (1969) was a nursing scholar whose writings proceeded from Frankl's work and recognized the shortcomings of competing psychotherapeutic approaches. She stated,

Those who should be able to assist the ill individual either cannot or do not know how to do so. And what can be more demoralizing to an ill individual than to believe that his illness and suffering are meaningless? The tragedy is that the problems are not even recognized by those whose responsibility is to help and comfort.

(p. 124)

She developed methods to assist patients to find "meaning in life." One strategy she used was called the parable method. Here she would impart a parable to a patient, which illustrated the point that no human being is exempt from illness. Such approaches used by proponents of Frankl try to impress on patients, who feel life is meaningless, that they have the ultimate choice in their attitude toward their illness. Key concepts in Travelbee's human-to-human relationship model are hope, suffering, and interaction.

Another proponent of Frankl's work, William Gould (1993), describes meaning analysis as having a focus "on the human spirit as the key resource for recapturing health wholeness and caring for the fully human person" (p. 152). He outlined phases of meaning making. These phases coincide with the Frankl's therapeutic approach. First is the general search for meaning, second is the discovery of a single important meaning, and third is the realization that many meaningful tasks are waiting.

Central to these phases is the spiritual dimension, which Gould asserts "is omitted from Freudian psychoanalysis, behavior therapy, reality therapy and gestalt therapy" (p. 152). Such approaches can assist patients to (1) gain distance from symptoms through "dereflection"; (2) modify their attitudes, which helps to reduce harmful symptoms; (3) become open to change; and (4) search for goals that will help in finding purpose and meaning.

This approach is congruent with a holistic nursing philosophy. The "therapy" of logotherapy revolves around the tenets of this perspective which are incorporated into the plan of care for persons whose lives are devoid of meaning. An example is biogenics, or a system of relaxation techniques for voluntary self-regulation. Self-identification exercises such as "Who Am I" are ways in which therapists can develop this self-discovery and, in turn, more fully help clients to find meaning in life.

In summary, this discussion of meaning began with the description of levels of meaning, and the literature focused mainly on the "meaning in life" level. Meaning has been described as (1) subjectively constructed, (2) culturally constructed, and (3) existentially derived from values connected to a spiritual dimension in which the "meaning of life" level is most explicit. To this point "meaning in life" is understood as what one takes from the world and what one gives to the world. Meaning making from a variety of perspectives places importance on the patient or the individual engaged in making meaning of living with chronic illness. The next section reviews current literature on meaning making.

Newer inductive ways of looking at meaning

A review of the literature from sociology, nursing, anthropology, and psychology revealed difficulty in distinguishing between the words experience and meaning. An analysis of this review reveals the common synonymous use of both terms, at times independent of any supporting theory or framework. There were sparse papers discussing meaning in chronic illness (Zucker, 1999). A Canadian nursing scholar (Rose, 1995) undertook a study to explore and describe meanings that families ascribe to the intensive care unit experience. All families identified initial meanings described as "It could go either way." Families who obtained positive cues from the patient went on to "Everything is good," while families who received negative cues from the staff proceeded to "Like living on a roller-coaster." The outcome of this investigation led the author to describe the meanings as correlated with the illness trajectories which were positive as "Going to make it" or negative as "There is no hope." Rose concluded that families' meanings changed over time, because of cues (stimuli from patients, staff, and the environment) used by families to assess their situation.

In another study, the meaning of illness for cancer patients was examined explicitly within the symbolic interactionist perspective (Fife, 1994). Conceptualization of meaning was influenced by the work of sociologist Peter Marris' (1974) work with loss and change. Marris described "structures of meaning," which refer to a basic aspect of human psychology. Structures of meaning are the "organized structures of understanding and emotional attachments, by which grown people interpret and assimilate their environment" (p. 4). A specific link was made between meaning and identity and that meaning is understood in terms of continuity between the past and the present. Meaning was operationally defined as "the individual's perception of the potential significance of an event, such as the occurrence of serious illness, for the self and one's plan of action" (Fife, p. 310). Meaning was conceptualized in relation to patients' adaptation to their cancer. Data was categorized in two dimensions, as self-meaning or contextual. Results from both studies are supported by the assumptions underlying symbolic interactionism in that patients, others, and the setting all influence meaning making.

An updated review of this literature discovered that there are fewer than 20 research studies examining the meaning of a chronic illness experience. The majority are focused on providing practitioners with tools to assist individuals and families to cope with issues emerging from chronic illness management, and to provide the chronically ill persons with avenues for positive meaning making. See Table 2.1 for a description of these studies.

Fourteen of 17 articles were dissertations and all focus on living with a chronic health problem and the meaning this has for the individual or family. Studies were mostly qualitative descriptive or non-experimental, using interviews and surveys as the primary sources of data collection. Findings

Table 2.1 Research on the meaning of chronic illness experiences

Study author	Title	Methodology	Data collection/Analysis	Results
M. A. Tarko (2003)	A grounded theory study of the experience of spirituality among persons living with schizophrenia	Ground theory	Interviews, focus groups	Engagement in self-care activities to achieve wellness
E. L. Weiss (2003)	A narrative-relational approach to grief therapy with a bereaved parent	Review of literature and case report	Interviews	Coping strategies emerged during psychotherapy
M. P. Mellors (1999)	IDS, self-transcendence, and quality of life (HIV, immune deficiency)	Descriptive cross-sectional study; grounded theory	Questionnaires and interviews	Using self-transcendence, individuals could make meaning of their lives
J. A. Riley (2022)	Exploring the emotional dimensions and coping processes of living with mitochondrial disease in emerging adulthood	Qualitative descriptive	Interviewing and narrative analysis	Coping such as using meaning centered affirmations
K. M. Glaser (2016)	Finding meaning through illness narratives: Latino perceptions of diabetes in a post-industrial American city	Qualitative descriptive	Interviews and surveys	Self-management education; enabling resources
C. A. Fruhauf (2007)	Grandchildren's perceptions of caring for grandparents	Qualitative descriptive	Semi-structured interviews	Developing coping measures to adapt to caregiving situations
Paterson et al. (1999)	Living with diabetes as a transformational experience	Grounded theory	A modified "think-aloud" technique, formal interviews, and final focus group interviews	Personal transformation and control in self-care decision-making

(Continued)

Table 2.1 (Continued)

Study author	Title	Methodology	Data collection/Analysis	Results
H.-M. Ho et al. (2016)	Living with illness and self-transcendence: The lived experience of patients with spinal muscular atrophy	Phenomenology	In-depth interviews	Self-transcendence to cope positively
M. S. Tijerina (2001)	Mexican-American women's perspectives of end-stage renal disease and the hemodialysis regimen: Psychosocial influences on compliance with treatment recommendations	Qualitative	Semi-structured in-depth interviews; medical record review	Overcoming compliance hampered by social determinants of health
J. Yepello (2011)	Psychological coping with breast cancer through prayer	Qualitative	Interviews	Prayer as a strategy to make meaning
M. A. Roush (2014)	The circle and the line: A transpersonal containment and integration process using the mandala and Neuro-Linguistic Programming (NLP) with individuals who experience severe and persistent mental illness and who are in crisis	Multiple case study	Pre-post questionnaires, interviews, and creating mandalas	Attainment of grace to find meaning in coping with chronic illness
H. B. Leibenberg (2009)	The impact of early traumatic experiences on bariatric patients: A qualitative exploration of their "voices"	Multiple case study	Case notes, written documents, reports, questionnaires, and information from the follow-up semi-structured interviews	Trauma-informed strategies to assist with coping and meaning making

Table 2.1 (Continued)

Study author	Title	Methodology	Data collection/Analysis	Results
M. R. Fraser (1999)	The meaning of care: Social support, informal caregiving, and HIV disease (immune deficiency)	Qualitative descriptive	In-depth interviews	Social support care giving networks enhanced meaning making
Lee et al. (2009).	The meaning of suffering in families: A human-becoming perspective	Qualitative descriptive exploratory study	Family member interviews	Education and support in coping stigma and finding meaning with decision-making
P.L. Cole (2004)	The stress process and chronic illness: Sickle cell disease and its impact on the performance of social roles and mental health among black women	Mixed methods	Surveys and interviews	Faith as social support in coping with chronic illness
M. N. Lewis (2010)	Transformative learning in the multiple sclerosis (MS) community: An ethnographic study examining how and in what ways transformative learning is realized and lived out among members of an MS community	Ethnography	Survey, interview	Transformative learning, coping with marginalization
S. N. Bailey (2016)	Working while living with chronic illness: A multiple case study of full-time, white-collar employees' experiences	Multiple case study	Interviews	Bring at work fostered meaning
H. O. Kim, and H. J. Kim (2020)	Experiences of inpatients living with lung cancer in South Korea	Grounded theory	In-depth interviews	Meaning making through effective care management

across all studies focused on how persons with chronic and often stigmatizing illnesses make meaning of living with their illnesses. Coping strategies, educational resources, and faith were necessary to support meaning making. Overcoming marginalization, stigma, and trauma were important themes described by researchers.

Summary

The historical review of philosophical perspectives has emphasized the importance of levels of meaning and a parallel is made between the assumptions of symbolic interactionism and these levels, particularly the meaning of people, things, and situations and the meaning of signs and symbols. Meaning becomes the description of the episode or the occurrence "at that time," within that setting, and because of some interaction with others. Changes in any of those variables change the meaning, or how the individual defines their situation. A new language is emerging from the contemporary literature in attempts to label meaning. Symbolic interactionism focuses on the meanings of things, events, and situations, or the level designated by Burbank, as meaning in life. According to symbolic interactionism, meaning is an entity which develops, changes, and is sustained across time. Symbolic interactionism ties experience to meaning, and that meaning is derived from experiences across time, interactions with others and the setting or environment. This is evident from the review of the literature and "meaning in life" is central to the discussion. While symbolic interactionism also asks questions about meaning on an existential level, for the most part meanings arise out of the concrete notions about interactions with others, symbols, and within social settings.

Conversely, the existential perspective, described by Frankl, purports that finding meaning in one's life does *not* depend on interaction to the same degree required of symbolic interactionism. Logotherapy, as a therapeutic approach, was developed to treat an "existential vacuum" common to persons who suffer meaningless lives. In this case, while the search for meaning may be central to life, finding meaning is not guaranteed; it cannot be assumed that meaning in life is the outcome of searching for it. A definition of meaning for Frankl's proponents refers mainly to "that which is meant." Because some contemporary therapists employing logotherapeutic methods equate meaningless in life with depression, perhaps emergence from depression is also equated with finding meaning.

This discussion seems particularly timely today, as there are growing health concerns about addiction, post-traumatic stress, and other mental health conditions. According to the Substance Abuse and Mental Health Services Administration (2023), over 22% of the 12 and older population have used illicit drugs within the year and 46% of young adults 18–25 had either a mental illness or substance-use disorder. We also know from the Adverse Childhood Experience (ACS) study there is a "graded relationship between the breadth of exposure to abuse or household dysfunction during childhood and multiple risk factors for several of the leading causes of death in adults" (Felitti et al., 1998, p. 245). These include ischemic heart disease, cancer, chronic lung disease, skeletal fractures, and liver disease. Taken together, social and psychological determinants of health require investigation and strategies that will assist persons to move from states of illness to states of health. This requires hard work on the part of the patient to make efforts in self-care such as practicing stress reduction, paying attention to healthy eating and maintaining healthy exercise and sleep. A challenge for healthcare providers, knowing that non-technological efforts at wellness may prove too hard for some individuals, requires providing support to increase and maintain patient motivation to change.

Nursing studies of meaning in chronic illness from 1999 forward have focused on shifting the paradigm of research traditions to include alternate modes of describing meaning and experience. These have mainly included qualitative descriptive methods examining the meaning of living with a chronic illness and strategies to support coping. In 1999, Sally Thorne outlined a discussion of the science of exploring this concept as a move toward knowledge construction. While not discarding traditional methods of research especially in delineating outcomes, the use of qualitative methods, such as case study, to uncover the subjective meaning of life experiences is equally important.

Meaning and experience are inextricably bound. Perspectives from symbolic interaction, social construction, and existentialism have provided frameworks from which approaches have been successful in eliciting meaning and providing trust, support, and motivation to persons engaged in change. The next chapter makes connections from these perspectives to the use of case study methodology.

References

Bailey, S. N. (2016). *Working while living with chronic illness: A multiple case study of full-time, white-collar employees' experiences* [Dissertation abstracts international]. ProQuest Information & Learning.

Balcar, K. (1995). Meaningfulness of life and personality. *Ceskoslovenska Psychologie, 39*(6), 496–502.

Becker, H. (1966). *Social problems. A modern approach*. John Wiley & Sons.

Berger, P. L., & Luckman, T. (1967). *The social construction of reality. A treatise in the sociology of knowledge*. Doubleday & Co.

Blumer, H. (1969). *Symbolic interactionism*. Prentice Hall.

Brown, J. A., & Romanchuk, B. J. (1994). Existential social work practice with the aged: Theory and practice. *Journal of Gerontological Social Work, 23*(1–2), 49–65.

Brown, P. (1991). Themes in medical sociology. *Journal of Health Politics, Policy, and Law, 16*(31), 595–604.

Burbank, P. (1988). *Meaning in life among older adults* [Unpublished doctoral dissertation]. Boston University.

Burbank, P. (1992). How meaning in life affects health status of older adults. *Gerontological Nursing, 18*(9), 19–28.

Calabrese, E. J. (1974). *The evolutionary basis of logotherapy* [Unpublished doctoral dissertation]. University of Massachusetts.

Charon, J. M. (1992). *Symbolic interactionism. An introduction, an interpretation, an integration.* Prentice Hall.

Cole, P. L. (2004). *The stress and process of chronic illness: Sickle cell disease and its impact on the performance of social roles and mental health among black women* [Dissertation abstracts international]. ProQuest Information & Learning.

Dubos, R. (1970). *Reason awake: Science for man.* Columbia University Press.

Fabry, J. B. (1968). *The pursuit of meaning: Logotherapy applied to life.* Beacon Press.

Felitti, V. J., Anda, R. F., Nordenberg, D., Williamson, D. F., Spitz, A. M., Edwards, V., Koss, M. P., & Marks, J. S. (1998). Relationship of childhood abuse and household dysfunction to many of the leading causes of death in adults. The adverse childhood experiences (ACE) study. *American Journal of Preventive Medicine, 14*(4), 245–258. https://doi.org/10.1016/s0749-3797(98)00017-8; PMID: 9635069

Fife, B. L. (1994). The conceptualization of meaning in illness. *Social Science & Medicine, 38*(21), 309–316.

Fisher, B., & Strauss, A. (1978). Interactionism. In T. Bottomore & R. Nisbet (Eds.), *A history of sociological analysis.* Basic Books.

Frankl, V. E. (1963). *Man's search for meaning: An introduction to logotherapy.* Simon & Shuster.

Frankl, V. E. (1969). *The will to meaning: Foundations and applications of logotherapy.* New American Library.

Fraser, M. R. (1999). *The meaning of care: Social support, informal caregiving and HIV disease (immune deficiency)* [Dissertation abstracts international]. ProQuest Information & Learning.

Fruhauf, C. A. (2007). *Grandchildren's perceptions of caring for grandparents* [Dissertation abstracts international]. ProQuest Information & Learning.

Glaser, K. M. (2016). *Finding meaning through illness narratives: Latino perceptions of diabetes in a post-industrial American city* [Dissertation abstracts international]. ProQuest Information & Learning.

Goffman, E. (1972). On face-work: An analysis of ritual elements in social interaction. In *Interaction ritual: Essays on face-to-face behaviour* (pp. 5–45). Penguin Books.

Good, B., & Good, M. D. (1982). Toward a meaning-centered analysis of popular illness categories: "Fright illness" and "heart distress". In A. J. Marsala & G. M. White (Eds.), *Cultural conceptions of mental health and therapy.* Kluwer.

Gould, W. B. (1993). *Viktor E. Frankl: Life with meaning.* Brooks/Cole Publishing.

Gove, P. B. (Ed.). (1986). *Webster's third new international dictionary.* Meriam Webster Inc.

Hanrahan, P. M. (1995). *The social construction of sexual harassment in nursing* [Unpublished dissertation]. The University of Massachusetts.

Harper, K. V. (1990). Meaning and midlife crisis: A logotherapy approach. *International Forum for Logotherapy*, *13*(1), 76–78.

Hilbert, R. A. (1984). The acultural dimensions of chronic pain: Flawed reality construction and the problem of meaning. *Social Problems*, *31*(4), 365–378.

Ho, H.-M., Tseng, Y.-M., Hsin, Y.-M., & Lin, W.-T. (2016). Living with illness and self-transcendence: The lived experience of patients with spinal muscular atrophy. *Journal of Advanced Nursing*, *72*(11), 2695–2705.

Hutzell, R. R. (1992). A values worksheet. *International Forum for Logotherapy*, *15*(1), 22–29.

Kim, H. O., & Kim, H. J. (2020). Experiences of inpatients living with lung cancer in South Korea. *Asian Oncology Nursing*, *20*(1), 28–38.

Kimble, M. A., Melvin, A., & Ellor, J. W. (1989). The use of meaning for the elderly. *International Forum for Logotherapy*, *12*(1), 59–61.

Kleinman, A. (1986). *Social origins of distress and disease*. Yale University Press.

Kleinman, A., Eisenberg, L., & Good, B. (1978). Culture, illness, and care. Clinical lessons from anthropologic and cross-cultural research. *Annals of Internal Medicine*, *88*(2), 251–258.

Kostis, J. B., Rosen, R. C., Brondolo, E., Taska, L., Smith, D. E., & Wilson, A. C. (1992). Superiority of nonpharmacologic therapy compared to propranolol and placebo in men with mild hypertension: A randomized prospective trial. *American Heart Journal*, *123*(2), 466–474.

Lantz, J. (1996). Logotherapy as trauma therapy. *Crisis Intervention and Time-Limited Treatment*, *2*(3), 243–253.

Lee, O. J., Choi, Y. S., & Doucet, T. J. (2009). The meaning of suffering in families. A human becoming perspective. *Nursing Science Quarterly*, *22*(2), 154–159.

Leibenberg, H. B. (2009). *The impact of early traumatic experiences on bariatric patients: A qualitative exploration of their 'voices'* [Dissertation abstracts international]. ProQuest Information & Learning.

Lewis, M. N. (2010). *Transformative learning in the multiple sclerosis (MS) community: An ethnographic study examining how and in what ways transformative learning is realized and lived out among members of an MS community* [Dissertation abstracts international]. ProQuest Information & Learning.

Lukas, E. (1991). Meaning-centered family therapy. *International Forum for Logotherapy*, *14*(2), 67–74.

Malone, R. E. (1995). Heavy users of emergency services: Social construction of a policy problem. *Social Science and Medicine*, *40*(4), 469–477.

Marris, P. (1974). *Loss and change*. Random House.

Mead, G. H. (1934). *Mind, self, and society from the standpoint of a social behaviorist*. University of Chicago Press.

Mellors, M. P. (1999). *AIDS, self-transcendence, and quality of life. (HIV, immune deficiency)* [Dissertation abstracts international]. ProQuest Information & Learning.

Ornish, D. (1990). *Dr. Dean Ornish's program for reversing heart disease*. Random House.

Paterson, B., Thorne, S., Crawford, J., & Tarko, M. (1999). *Living with diabetes as a transformational experience* [Dissertation abstracts international]. ProQuest Information & Learning.

Riley, J. A. (2022). *Exploring the emotional dimensions and coping processes of living with mitochondrial disease in emerging adulthood* [Dissertation abstracts international]. ProQuest Information & Learning.

Rose, P. A. (1995). The meaning of critical illness to families. *Canadian Journal of Nursing Research, 27*(4), 83–87.

Roush, M. A. (2014). *The circle and the line: A transpersonal containment and integration process using the mandala and neuro-linguistic programming (NLP) with individuals who experience severe and persistent mental illness and who are in crisis* [Dissertation abstracts international]. ProQuest Information & Learning.

Sadiq, I. Z. (2023). Lifestyle medicine as a modality for prevention and management of chronic diseases. *Journal of Taibah University Medical Science, 18*(5), 1115–1117. https://doi.org/10.1016/j.jtumed.2023.04.001; PMID: 37187803; PMCID: PMC10176046

Sarbin, T. R., & Kitsuse, J. I. (1994). *Constructing the social.* Sage Publications.

Schneider, J. (1985). Social problems theory: The constructionist view. *American Review of Sociology, 11*, 209–229.

Schutz, A. (1967). *Phenomenology of the social world.* Northwestern University Press.

Spector, M., & Kitsuse, J. (1987). *Constructing social problems.* Aldine De Gruyter.

Spradley, J. (1979). *The ethnographic interview.* Holt, Rinehart & Winston, Inc.

Starck, P. L. (1992). Suffering in a nursing home: Losses of the human spirit. *International Forum for Logotherapy, 15*(2), 76–79.

Strauss, A. (1971). *The context of social mobility.* Aldine De Gruyter.

Substance Abuse and Mental Health Services Administration. (2023). *SAMHSA announces national survey and drug use and health (NSDUH) results detailing mental illness and substance use levels in 2021.* SAMHSA. https://www.samhsa.gov/newsroom/press-announcements/20230104/samhsa-announces-nsduh-results-detailing-mental-illness-substance-use-levels-2021

Tarko, M. A. (2003). *A grounded theory study of the experience of spirituality among persons living with schizophrenia* [Dissertation abstracts international]. ProQuest Information & Learning.

Thorne, S. (1999). The science of meaning in chronic illness. *International Journal of Nursing Studies, 36*(5), 397–404.

Tijerina, M. S. (2001). *Mexican-American women's perspectives of end-stage renal disease and the hemodialysis regimen: Psychosocial influences on compliance with treatment recommendations* [Dissertation abstracts international]. ProQuest Information & Learning.

Travelbee, J. (1969). *Intervention in psychiatric nursing.* F.A. Davis Company.

Turner, J. H. (1991). *The structure of sociological theory* (5th ed.). Wadsworth Publishing Co.

Wadsworth, T. M. (1992). Logotherapy and the 12 step programs in the treatment of substance abuse. *International Forum for Logotherapy*, *15*(1), 13–21.

Weiss, E. L. (2003). *A narrative-relational approach to grief therapy with a bereaved parent* [Dissertation abstracts international]. ProQuest Information & Learning.

Yepello, J. (2011). *Psychological coping with breast cancer through prayer* [Dissertation abstracts international]. ProQuest Information & Learning.

Zucker, D. M. (1999). *Two contrasting cases of men's experiences with chronic coronary heart disease post 1985* [Unpublished doctoral dissertation]. University of Rhode Island.

3 Case study methodology

Donna M. Zucker, Patricia Bruckenthal, and Miki Patterson

Historical overview of case study method

The earliest use of case study method seemed to have been in psychiatry and later spread to medicine and clinical psychology (Bromley, 1986; Bolgar, 1965). Bolgar notes, "it is the traditional approach to all clinical research, is essentially exploratory in nature, focuses on the individual, and it aims primarily at discovering and generating hypotheses" (p. 28). The original purpose for using case study was to find a solution to the person's problem. According to Bromley (1986), administrative reports, military and technical reports, and particularly judiciary inquiries were probably among the earliest branches of knowledge to employ case studies. The case study can take many forms:

> a summary statement in ordinary language, a detailed technical report containing scientific and professional concepts and data, a judicial or quasi-judicial report (like a barrister presents his client's case in a court of law), a computerized catalogue of information, a documentary film, and so on.
>
> (p. 1)

Bromley (1986) has used this method to study the individual person, usually in a problematic situation, and for a relatively short period of time. This period, he considers, is a segment of life history. In this study, this notion was somewhat extended as it was found that life events were so integral to the journey. Early times in participants' lives were referred to and explored further to understand things that were said.

At the turn of the century, at about the same time that the method was being developed in medicine, psychiatry, and psychoanalytic research, an independent branch of case study research concerned itself with child psychology, sociology, and anthropology (Bolgar, 1965). In the early twentieth century, nonmedical evidence of case studies was documented in the diaries of investigators in the area of child development and psychology. Bolgar goes on to claim that the early sociologists' use of "life history" (personal documents

DOI: 10.4324/9781003435358-3

about a person's life) is another example of case study, though they did not use that term: "the questions they asked were in essence not too different from those of the clinicians" (p. 29).

By the mid-century, case study method turned to the study of aging, creative individuals, death, and suicide. While the issues of etiology have always been of interest to clinical psychology, an interest grew in researchers using the case study method. They turned their attention to the area of what was coined "psychotherapeutic interaction" (Bolgar, p. 30), where the aim of study is the interactional process between two people, which is designed to produce a change in one of them. In conclusion, Bolgar emphasized that despite the various forms of and purposes for using case studies, case study research must "study the entire case."

Methodology

Case studies have different purposes and methods compared with other research designs and are rooted in psychology and sociology. Nurses are interested in examining a human being's life experiences using a holistic approach, thus their research is well suited to strategies from both traditions. This is in line with Yin's (1994) description of the methodology as a preferred design when examining contemporary events when relevant behaviors cannot be manipulated. Boundaries between the context and phenomena are not demarcated. Finally, the case study can use multiple sources of data for a full understanding of the phenomena. Fishman's (1999) pragmatic approach underscores the holistic assessment and analysis of individual components and the interrelationships between them. Recently he emphasized the need for rigor and definition for clinical/applied psychology, and that pragmatic case study includes mixed methods (Fishman, 2016). According to Stake (1995), case studies aim to fully understand the case or the phenomenon often resulting in constructed meanings and naturalistic generalizations.

Generating meaning

An important activity is to craft useful approaches to collect meaningful data. Miles and Huberman (1994) have described 13 tactics for generating meaning from qualitative data. Such tactics range from descriptive to explanatory and from concrete to abstract (see Table 3.1). According to Miles and Huberman, the first three tactics tell us "what goes with what." The next two tell us "what's there." The next two help "sharpen our understanding." The next four help us "see things and their relationships more abstractly." Finally the last two help us to "assemble a coherent understanding of the data" (pp. 245–246). It may not be necessary to use all these tactics in any one case study (Zucker, 2001).

Table 3.1 Strategies to generate meaning

What goes with what	Noting patterns	Clustering	Seeing plausibility	
What's there	Making metaphors	Counting		
Sharpen our understanding	Making comparisons	Partitioning variables		
See things and their relationships more abstractly	Subsuming particulars into the general	Factoring	Noting relations between variables	Finding intervening variables
Assemble a coherent understanding of the data	Building a logical chain of evidence	Making conceptual/ theoretical coherence		

Source: Adapted from Miles & Huberman (1994)

Rationale for using case study methodology

Case study was the method used in Zucker's study of men with chronic heart disease (2001). The main focus of that study was fully describing and understanding the case. Additionally, the method fit well with the intent of the research questions which were aimed at eliciting description and meaning, particularly across a long period of adult life. This method was congruent with the theoretical foundations of symbolic interactionism and existential analysis. The major source of data was interviews. Emphasis and importance were placed on the interview data because the research questions were aimed at eliciting the client's perspective and to capture the essence of the experience of living with heart disease. All other data (medical records, spouse and nurse interviews) were used as a way to support, add to, or to identify potentially conflicting information from the interview data.

Case study method also allowed for the development of the researcher as a biographer. According to Stake (1995), "the chronology of life is explored against a thematic network," for example, a set of issues. In this, the biographer knows that to portray the occurrences in life across time is crucial to the development of understanding the complexities of human life. What emerges are concepts, themes, patterns, and phrases which are unique to the individual's experiences. The significance of this method lies in its importance to experiential understanding, and as a basis for naturalistic generalization. Naturalistic generalization is a form of generalization, not scientific induction, "arrived at by recognizing the similarities of objects and issues in and out of context and by sensing the natural covariations of happenings" (Stake, 1978, p. 6). This study focused on the experiences of patients with chronic health problems mainly through in-depth interviews. An emphasis was placed on describing the trajectory of chronic illness across time. The intent behind this was not to focus on the patient's "life history," although the patient's experiences of wellness and illness were viewed within the context of each patient's entire life.

Focus of analysis

Both Stake and Yin have devised analytic techniques that have informed Zucker's case study design and analysis. Major themes were identified with the use of maps and typologies that emerged as focal areas of the analysis. The metaphor "journey" became a central organizing concept, and was linked to a variety of subconcepts, and relationships among them were sought. This study described two contrasting cases and each was analyzed separately with an eye toward describing experience and meaning. According to Feigin et al.'s (1991) description, one appeared as a "normal" case and one an "extreme" case. The strategy was to focus the analysis on each individual's journey by concentrating on how it: (1) was tied to a physiologic state, (2) carried consequences, and (3) was compared with the typical trajectory. After describing experience, describing meaning, and discovering the focus of the analysis, a study protocol emerged (see Table 3.2). While this protocol differs only slightly from those in the literature, differences reflect the specificity required in this nursing study.

Table 3.2 Protocol for the case study

Purpose and rationale for case study	Significance of the phenomena of interest	Research questions			
Design based on the unit of analysis and research purpose					
Data collection and management techniques	Field methods	Transcribed notes and interviews	Mapping of major concepts	Building typologies	Member checking
Describe the full case	In depth interviews of individual	Chart review	Interview significant others	Interview spouses	Interview care givers
Focus the analysis built on themes linked to purpose and unit of analysis					
Analyze findings based on the purpose, rationale, and research questions	Patient's perspective	Nursing perspective	Cross-case comparison	Write up the case from an emic perspective	Biography, autobiography and narratives
Establishing rigor	Credibility	Transferability	Dependability	Confirmability	

Source: Adapted from Zucker (2001)

Comparison of case study styles

Bruckenthal (2001) examined the characteristics of case study and to explore meaning in context. In characterizing case study, this method begins with a priori propositions regarding the development of theory but is not useful for scientific (statistical) generalization. Instead, a goal of case study is analytic generalization, and to expand or generalize theories (Yin, 1994). Stake (1995) addresses generalization in terms of the emergence of certain activities, problems, or responses that come up time and time again during the case study process. Generalizations about these situations can be drawn from the data and then refined to gain an understanding of the situation. Most significantly this methodology provides for the examination of the meaning and understanding of contemporary phenomena. Table 3.3 outlines a comparison of three case study researchers' processes using a framework developed by Mariano (2001).

While there are pros and cons to using case study method, the overall assessment is that it remains an invaluable strategy for increasing knowledge and understanding human beings. Mariano (2001) summarized that the pros of using case study research far outweigh the cons. Case studies are significant, complete, and compelling and include the participant at every step (Yin, 1994).

Case study methodology use in nursing research – 2003–2017

The results of three integrative reviews of using case study methodology in nursing, from three countries and completed across 14 years are presented here.

Integrative review one

The first integrative review (Patterson, 2003) examined nursing research that used case study methodology. Inclusion criteria included articles that were peer-reviewed, were nursing research articles, published from 1995 to 2003, and available in English. Data were assembled by author, year, purpose, design, focus, sample, analysis, findings, rigor, and research recommendations. Of the 67 citations retrieved, 41 were obtained, and 35 studies met inclusion criteria. Studies were analyzed and the key findings are summarized in Table 3.4.

Patterson (2003) summarized her findings according to a data collection tool based on guidelines of Jackson (1980) and Ganong (1987). Across the 35 studies reviewed, it was clear nursing needed to have its own case study protocol based on nursing science. Analysis of studies reviewed most reported meaning from the patient's perspective, used multiple cases for analysis, and

Table 3.3 Comparison of three case study research processes

Framework elements	Stake (1995)	Yin (1994)	Fishman (1999, 2016)
Purpose and Questions	Etic vs. emic issues	Ask how and why questions	Interpretive hermeneutic vs. pragmatic paradigms
Theoretical Framework Unit of Analysis	Issues as conceptual structure The "case" A specific person, program, institution A bounded system focused on object vs. process	Literature, tied to propositional statements Persons events, organizational programs "Who" or "what" parts of the system with time boundaries having a beginning and end to the case	Holistic, systems oriented: roadmap Individuals from many points of view, including their internal subjective life, their personalities, their overtly observable behaviors, and the historical and contemporary contexts of their lives Boundaries are detailed and express why they were chosen
Study Design	Triangulation protocols	2×2 matrix of four designs: single holistic, single embedded multiple holistic and multiple embedded. Meet criteria for logical adequacy	Holistic or single unit vs. embedded or multiple units of analysis Meet criteria for logical adequacy
Data Sources	Observation, interviewing, document reviews	Multiples sources of evidence: documentation, archival records, interviews, direct observation, participant observation and physical artifacts	Participant observation and use qualitative and quantitative measures
Analysis	Pattern matching Naturalistic generalizations refer to study results that can be generalized to a broader theory	Pattern matching: how the overall pattern of results matched the predicted one; if so, internal validity is strengthened External validity is termed analytical generalization	Pattern matching Analysis of similar cases in multiple series to see if a pattern emerges more than once; cross-case analysis and qualitative meta-analysis
Writing the Report/ Interpretation	Should occur early in the study, follow specific guidelines, use narrative text as illustration	Should occur early in the study, follow specific guidelines, use narrative text as illustration	Should occur early in the study, follow specific guidelines, use narrative text as illustration

Source: Adapted from Mariano (2001)

Table 3.4 Summary analysis of nursing studies using case study method (n=35)

Focus	Wide focus
Definition	37% of studies did not define case
Purpose	67% describe the case
Ethics	All but 1 mentioned ethical approval of study
Unit of Analysis	37% event or role; 32% individual
Design	65% collective case study, 21% instrumental and 13% intrinsic
Sample	66% multiple cases, 30% single cases and 2 embedded cases. 75% had <8 participants
Data Collection Sources	Multiple sources: 88% face to face interviews; 60% field notes and/or observations; 60% viewed documents
Analysis	Written in the participant's perspective (46%), nursing perspective (13%), and institution's perspective (11%) or as example of teaching case (11%). Computer-aided analysis was reported as using NUD*IST (6%), SPSS (3%), and Ethnograph (6%) software programs.
Research question	90% of studies analyzed based on research question
Voice	46% written in the participant's perspective; 13% in nursing perspective
Technical aided analysis	Computer-aided analysis 15%
Meaning making strategies	97% looked for patterns; plausibility 2%; making metaphors 11%; counting 20%; making comparisons 63%; partitioning variables 31%
Other analytic strategies	Subsuming particular to general 30%; factoring 9%; noting relationships between variables 34%; identifying intervening variables 9%
Rigor	Prolonged engagement used in 63% of the studies. Researchers almost unanimously utilized *triangulation* of data (43%) and method (46%) or combination. Peer debriefing (29%), negative case (3%), member checking (40%), audit trail (80%), descriptive vividness (93%) were apparent.
Referential adequacy	All studies used a recording device(s) for interviews and focus groups; 63% prolonged engagement; nearly all used triangulation of data; 43% triangulation of data and method; 46% a combination; 29% peer debriefing; 3% negative case; 40% member checking; 80 audit trail and 93% descriptive vividness.
Findings	93% demonstrated conceptual or theoretical connections used to compare and contrast findings.
Limitations	75% discussed study limitations and bias; 40% had recommendations for future research, although all contained conclusions in terms of nursing practice, policy recommendations or future care.

rigor in their analyses. Additionally, her findings revealed that the experts having the most influence on nursing studies have been Yin (2014) and Stake (1995). It is also clear that case study was not well defined and still in its early stages of use in nursing.

Table 3.5 Summary analysis of nursing studies using qualitative case study method (QCSM) (n=41)

Where has QCSM been used in nursing research?	Studied populations across the age continuum and in a cross section of nursing contexts, including institutions and communities. Most of the studies were in acute care and community public health (15 of 41).
Why has QCSM been used in nursing research?	To describe, explore, understand, and evaluate phenomenon of interest to nursing.
How has QCSM been used in nursing research?	Scoring of authenticity and methodological quality scored (1 low, 3 high) for explicit and 0 if implicit. 95% of the studies reviewed had moderate to high authenticity. Informational value was correlated to authenticity scores. 33% of studies did not mention strategies to promote methodological rigor.
How has QCSM use in nursing research been reported in the literature?	All published in peer-reviewed nursing and healthcare journals.

Source: Adapted from Anthony and Jack (2009)

Integrative review two

Another integrative review was completed in 2009 (Anthony & Jack, 2009) using Whittemore and Knafl's (2005) guideline for integrative review method and analysis. Forty-two papers from six databases from 2005 to 2007 were retrieved that met the eligibility criteria for analysis. The aims of the review were to critically analyze what is known about contemporary use of case study method in nursing research. Nine subgroups based on patient characteristics or context were further analyzed numerically and textually, and rated as to authenticity, methodological quality, and informational value. Data were synthesized evaluating study characteristics, data reduction, and comparison. Four research questions were posed, and summary responses can be viewed in Table 3.5.

This review revealed case study as a legitimate qualitative research method. It also emphasized the capacity of case study research to give voice to the otherwise unheard. Finally, this review concluded the method is consistent with nursing values such as holism and human caring. The authors hoped this method would continue to be used in a rigorous way thus contributing to nursing knowledge and science.

Integrative review three

In 2017, de Andrade et al. completed an integrative review of using case study method in nursing. Multiple data bases were searched between 2010 and 2015, and of the 624 studies found, 50 met inclusion criteria and 92% were excluded because they did not apply a methodology. The study design was based on the Statement for Reporting Systematic Reviews and Meta-Analyses

Table 3.6 Categorization of articles based on nursing work process

Nurse education/care (n=12)	Nurse training, curricular development, pedagogical practices, teacher experience, and patient experience in nurse training
Care and management (n=29)	Nursing care practices in a variety of patient care areas; protocols in nursing care, models of health-care service provision, and the impact of nurses' performance
Administration (n=8)	Care management, nursing workload, nursing care planning, organizational and extra-organizational factors

Source: Adapted from de Andrade et al. (2017)

of Studies Guidelines and Preferred Reporting Items for Systematic Reviews and Meta-Analyses (PRISMA) checklist. A protocol was developed by the authors that guided data collection. Studies were categorized as nursing care, nursing education, and administration. Eighty percent used the methodology of Yin versus 20% using that of Stake. See Table 3.6 for these categorizations.

Andrade et al. (2017) concluded the case study papers mainly using the methods of Yin and Stake, with Stake's method used the most in studies of nursing education. The use of this methodology in nursing was applicable to all areas of nursing practice and administration, offering a variety of data sources, studying both single and multiple cases. Uppermost in their evaluation was that the researcher must first determine the appropriateness of the case study to the phenomenon of interest, use a planning protocol and detailed data collection and analyses procedures.

Summary

The integrative reviews have confirmed earlier findings of the usefulness of case study research in nursing. Established methodologists such as Yin and Stake have informed the majority of nursing case studies. Accurate protocols and strategies are well established in the literature and form a basis for continued use of this method in examining nursing phenomena, not easily understood using other research methods. A research protocol is essential in completing a rigorous and comprehensive case study. Finally, the close tie between philosophy, framework, and analysis is consistent with nursing's focus on human beings, and the meaning attributed to the events in their lives. The following chapter discusses trajectories of health and illness and the importance of describing these in case study research.

References

Anthony, S., & Jack, S. (2009). Qualitative case study methodology in nursing research: An integrative review. *Journal of Advanced Nursing, 65*(6), 1171–1181. https://doi.org/10.1111/j.1365-2648.2009.04998.x

Bolgar, H. (1965). The case study method. In B. B. Wolman (Ed.), *The handbook of clinical psychology* (pp. 28–38). McGraw Hill.

Bromley, D. B. (1986). *The case-study method in psychology and related disciplines.* John Wiley & Sons.

Bruckenthal, P. (2001). *A comparative look at contemporary case study methods* [Unpublished manuscript]. University of Massachusetts.

de Andrade, S. R., Ruoff, A. B., Piccoli, T., Schmitt, M. D., Ferreira, A., & Ammon Xavier, A. C. (2017). Case study as a nursing research method: An integrative review. *Texto & Contexto Enfermagem, 26*(4), e5360016. https://doi.org/10.1590/0104-07072017005360016

Feigin, J. R., Orum, A. M., & Sjoberg, G. (1991). *A case for case study.* The University of North Carolina Press.

Fishman, D. B. (1999). *The case for pragmatic psychology.* New York University Press.

Fishman, D. B. (2016). The pragmatic case study in psychotherapy: A mixed methods approach informed by psychology's striving for methodological quality. *Clinical Social Work Journal, 45,* 238–252. https://doi.org/10.1007/s10615-016-0612-3

Ganong, L. H. (1987). Integrative reviews of nursing research. *Research in Nursing & Health, 10,* 1–11.

Jackson, G. (1980). Methods for integrative reviews. *Review of Educational Research, 50*(3), 438–460.

Mariano, C. (2001). Case study: The method. In P. Munhall & C. Boyd (Eds.), *Nursing research: A qualitative perspective.* Jones and Bartlett Publishers.

Miles, M. B., & Huberman, A. M. (1994). *Qualitative data analysis* (2nd ed.). Sage Publications.

Patterson, M. (2003). *How is case study methodology utilized in contemporary nursing research? An integrative research review* [Unpublished manuscript]. University of Massachusetts.

Stake, R. E. (1978). The case study method in social inquiry. *Educational Researcher, 7*(2), 5–8.

Stake, R. E. (1995). *The art of case research.* Sage Publications.

Whittemore, R., & Knafl, K. (2005). The integrative review: Updated methodology. *Journal of Advanced Nursing, 52*(5), 546–553.

Yin, R. K. (1994). *Case study research design and methods.* Sage Publications.

Yin, R. K. (2014). *Case study research design and methods* (5th ed.). Sage Publications.

Zucker, D. M. (2001). Using case study methodology in nursing. *The Qualitative Report, 6*(2), 1–13. https://doi.org/10.46743/2160-3715/2001.2002

4 Trajectories of health and illness

Donna M. Zucker and Sheila Pennell

Over the last 40 or more years there has been a growing interest in illness trajectory and the meaning that has for human beings, their lives, and families. In (Corbin, 1991), the *Journal Scholarly Inquiry for Nursing Practice* devoted an issue to the Corbin and Strauss Chronic Illness Trajectory Framework Model and asked several researchers to illustrate the fit between their research and this model. The articles addressed several chronic diseases. Authors summarized that trajectories are not always downward ending in death, are not about just about the illness but a context, and finally the model has an emphasis on prevention and is not exclusive to every specific disease. In 1998, Corbin published an update to keep in step with the changing healthcare environment, changing nursing care roles and the increasing number of persons living with chronic illness. The goals of the update were to propose a more streamlined model that is problem oriented using the nursing process. The nurse determines the biopsychosocial data that is needed and determines a "phase" of the current patient trajectory. Following the steps of the nursing process the nurse creates a plan of care, executes it, and evaluates the effectiveness of the plan. Model authors used this guiding framework to shape management strategies for their patients.

Continued interest in health trajectories emerged in 2011 when the journal *Nursing Research* devoted a supplement to health trajectory research. In that issue was a call for person-centered nursing science that underscores how much emphasis on the person must be instilled in the nursing curricula and practice for the future of healthcare. Henley et al. (2011) outlined a health trajectory research agenda that included four major areas: building the science for nursing research, developing a community of scientists in nursing, leveraging innovation and emerging areas of nursing research, and translating health trajectory research into findings across the life span and continuum of care (pp. 5–6).

During the 2000s, exploratory centers were funded by the NINR to look for solutions to assist patients and families adapt to heath trajectories. The University of Minnesota's Center for Health Trajectory research, funded by the NINR, supported 16 studies from 2005 to 2011 (Wyman, 2011). The aims

DOI: 10.4324/9781003435358-4

were to test interventions that, among other outcomes, would impact health trajectories of the clients and some studies looked at the determinants of health trajectories in several patient groups using a wide range of observational and experimental research approaches (Wyman & Henley, 2011). Adapting to the changing healthcare landscape, it is a linear model illustrating how health challenges are influenced by policies and interventions as well as access to quality healthcare, impacting the health outcome.

Duke University's A.D.A.P.T. Center used an industry model of leadership (Heifetz et al., 2009) to work with families adapting to health trajectories in both technical and adaptive domains. Their model was tested in several areas of nursing from the individual to the systems levels and involves the ever-changing health trajectory. The theory is that individuals adapt within the environment. They and their caregivers develop a strategy for care guided by the nurse leader. In terms of technical challenges, with knowledge and expertise a technical intervention may be required to solve the problem (Bailey et al., 2012). In the case of the adaptive challenge a complex problem occurs with no known solution requiring learning and behavior change requiring self-care and adopting new behaviors to resolve the challenge. Educational strategies are key to assisting patients and care givers with tools to improve health outcomes.

Middle range theory (Mishel, 1988), models of health behavior (Rolland, 1994) and self-care theories of chronic illness (Riegel et al., 2012) have emerged across the decades to assist nursing in the care planning of persons and families with chronic illness. As nursing continues to build a knowledge base in this area the work must keep pace with the changes in not only nursing and healthcare systems, but our world, cultures, and societies as well.

Functional measures and trajectory

The literature in this area has demonstrated that objective measures of functional status do not always correspond to a person's perceived functional status (Zucker, 2003). This perspective comes from the idea that despite the level of measured functional capacity by objective measures, persons often have their own view of functional reality. This is based in their explanatory model of illness and wellness and often is impacted by early life decision-making patterns (experience). For example, an elder's functional capacity can be assessed by objective measures of balance, endurance, gait, and self-report on quality of life. Taken together these comprise the health trajectory. Self-report is a temporal condition and refers to the day-to-day changes in persons' lives, as opposed to the fixed time of an objective measurement. In this sense, functional capacity refers to an individual's capability, under controlled conditions, to perform tasks and activities that are necessary or desirable in their lives. In Table 4.1, you can see a schema for health trajectory that brings together the temporal perception of the patient with functional status across time.

Table 4.1 Health trajectory

Functional capacity			
High			
Low	Phase 1	Phase 2	Phase 3

Phase 1. Early diagnosis, treatment, and return to baseline
Phase 2. Cycling in and out of treatment
Phase 3. Long-term chronic illness

If functional status is on the Y axis, and time is on the X axis, time can be described in terms of phases. Phase one is characterized as early in the diagnosis and treatment ending in discharge, cure, or complete recovery. Phase two is a period of cycling in and out of treatment, and phase three is a period of long-term chronic illness or post-traumatic experiences (Zucker, 1999). These phases correspond to functional capacity but are not necessarily linear.

In contrasting trajectories of patients with chronic hepatitis C (CHC) and chronic heart disease (CHD), it was found that in CHD, phase one is short, phase two can be very long with subtle decline and in phase three there may be an increase in unpleasant symptoms and decline. However, in CHC, there is a long quiescent phase one with no symptoms no signs. Once diagnosed in phase two, there is a very short and often one time only for optimal treatment that results in cure, relapse, or non-response. Phase three is long-term chronic illness until death, which may be precipitous or not depending on many factors (Zucker, 2003). Parsing typical from atypical trajectories assists in providing appropriate care at the appropriate time. Determining objective functional status as well as perceived functional status are both important components of the health trajectory.

Aging and health trajectory

Pennell (2011) undertook a case study as part of a concept analysis of successful aging. This case provides a poignant clinical example of a participant whose objectively measured functional capacity and subjective reports of well-being were contrasting. The analysis identified examples of Flood's (2003, 2005) theoretical work asserting successful aging consists of functional status, gerotranscendence, and spirituality, contributing to life satisfaction, which together lead to successful aging. In this case study narratives revealed three dimensions of successful aging. First was the participant's fierce independence, second a personal feeling about a force greater than oneself, and lastly an awareness of and choices that compensate for age-related losses.

At 96 years of age this participant was most likely in Phase three of her life trajectory. Objectively, rheumatoid arthritis significantly limited mobility and functional status. The participant had used a motorized chair for mobility for many years and required hands on assistance to rise from bed. The chronic illnesses and limitations had been present for many years without improvement. She reported a recent additional diagnosis of asthma causing difficulty breathing, improved with treatment. While objective measures of her functional status would have been rated as low (with dependence noted in many activities of daily living (ADL) tasks and nearly all instrumental or complex ADL tasks), her subjective, self-reported success was very high. Her narrative of self included a strong sense of meaning and purpose in her life, a small number of meaningful relationships a, enjoyment of solitude, reverence for plants and the natural world, a positive and affective position and effective prior planning. These elements are in strong congruence with Flood's model. She described her adaptative choices and supports of healthcare providers and home nursing as facilitators to her ongoing ability to function living alone at home.

Mapping trajectory

The trajectory of the illness or wellness can be mapped, including the inter-relationships of functional status, psychosocial, and spiritual needs. Common interventions for chronic illnesses are mainly pharmaceutical but more recently acceptance is growing for integrating mindfulness and relationship-centered strategies into the plan of care. Across 15 years of studying patient experiences and using case method to fully describe and understand chronic illness phenomena, a model of work emerged that framed completed research. The research trajectory can be envisioned as being composed of four major constructs. The upper left quadrant depicts the temporality of certain chronic conditions. In the upper right are strategies that describe from the individual's perspective, living with a chronic condition. In the lower right quadrant are objective measures that may be used to examine health and illness trajectory. In the lower left quadrant are the four dimensions that frame functional status across the illness trajectory. Circular arrows in the center illustrate the ongoing interaction and relationship of these four model constructs.

While the role of the nurse or care provider is absent from this model it is assumed that self-care and clinical partnership are key to healthy trajectory work. The importance of the day-to-day lived experience and the meaning that holds for the individual is significant. Thus, research using the case study research method is an excellent fit with trajectory work.

Recent trajectory research has supported expanding and/or incorporating existing models. Schoon and Krumwiede (2022) developed a holistic health determinants model based in socioecological theory. It aims to prepare users to take actions to improve health equity (p. 1070). This model also incorporates the lived experiences of persons across the lifespan and illustrates the intersecting relationships as well as the ecological influences on persons and communities and points out the importance of incorporating the social and physical environments into the assessment of lived experience. Sadly, the social and physical environmental health determinants representing 50% of the impact on health outcomes are seldom addressed (Schoon & Krumwiede, 2022). As healthcare has moved into a health promotion/disease prevention mode, our research must keep pace with the lived experiences of patients and intervene early in their health and illness trajectories. Chapter 5 focuses on self-care management.

References

Bailey, D. E., Docherty, S. L., Adams, J. A., Carthron, D. L., Corazzini, K., Day, J. R, Neglia, E., Thygeson, M., & Anderson, R. A. (2012). Studying the clinical encounter with the adaptive leadership framework. *Journal of Healthcare Leadership, 4.* https://doi.org/10.2147/JHL.S32686

Corbin, J. M. (1998). The Corbin and Strauss chronic illness trajectory model: An update. *Scholarly Inquiry for Nursing Practice: An International Journal, 12*(1), 33–41.

Corbin, J. M., & Strauss, A. (1991). A nursing model for chronic illness management based upon the trajectory framework. *Scholarly Inquiry for Nursing Practice, 5*(3). https://doi.org/10.1891/0889-7182.5.3.155

Flood, M. (2003). Successful aging: A concept analysis. *The Journal of Theory Construction & Testing, 6*(2), 105–108.

Flood, M. (2005). A mid-range nursing theory of successful aging. *The Journal of Theory Construction & Testing, 9*(2), 35–39.

Heifetz, R., Grashow, A., & Linsky, M. (2009). *The practice of adaptive leadership.* Harvard Business Press.

Henley, S. J., Wyman, J. F., & Gaugler, J. E. (2011). Health trajectory research: A call to action for nursing science. *Nursing Research, 60*(suppl 3), S79–S82.

Mishel, M. H. (1988). Uncertainty in illness. *Image: Journal of Nursing Scholarship, 20*, 225–232.

Pennell, S. (2011). *Successful aging at home* [Unpublished manuscript]. University of Massachusetts.

Riegel, B., Jaarsma, T., & Strömberg, A. (2012). A middle-range theory of self-care of chronic illness. *Advances in Nursing Science, 35*(3), 194–204.

Rolland, J. S. (1994). *Families, illness, and disability: An integrative treatment model.* Basic Books.

Schoon, P. M., & Krumwiede, K. (2022). A holistic health determinants model for public health nursing education and practice. *Public Health Nursing, 39*, 1070–1077.

Wyman, J. F. (2011). Overview of the center for health trajectory research. *Nursing Research, 60*(suppl 3), S83–S84.

Wyman, J. F., & Henley, S. J. (2011). Advancing nursing science through health trajectory research. An introduction. *Nursing Research, 60*(suppl 3), S1–S4.

Zucker, D. M. (1999). *Two contrasting cases of men's experiences with chronic coronary heart disease post 1985* [Unpublished doctoral dissertation]. University of Rhode Island.

Zucker, D. M. (2003). Relapse in hepatitis C: A case study. *Clinical Excellence for Nurse Practitioners, 7*(3), 53–59.

5   Self-care management

Donna M. Zucker, Annette Maruca,
Sonya LaChance, and Kimberly Dion

Defining self-care management

As people age, both multiple chronic conditions and disability rise (Iezzoni, 2010). People living with chronic conditions do so in their communities, with only brief periods spent in healthcare institutions. Thus, managing and caring becomes a role for the patient and the person(s) in their lives. In Chapter 4, the trajectory model of Corbin and Strauss outlined types of "work" done in managing chronic conditions and referred to them as a wellness trajectory. These are illness work, everyday life work, and biographical work (1985, p. 224). In this chapter self-care management is viewed as the work an individual with chronic illness does to maintain their health within a social context(s) and among social relationships.

Nursing self-care management

Several self-management theories have been developed across the past 60 years with many in the past 20. Of these, models put forth by Corbin and Strauss (1991) based on the chronic illness trajectory framework and Dorothy Orem's self-care deficit theory (2001) are the most widely described and tested in nursing. Self-care management, if begun early in life, establishes a norm for persons to be responsible for their health and to collaborate with the healthcare team to prevent illness and maintain wellness. In 2013, the National Institute of Nursing Research (NINR) convened a chronic illness group (Grady & Gough, 2014). They recommended areas of focus and approaches to self-care management that included: to use a standardized language, to expand several key areas of research, to use a multidisciplinary methods approach for future studies, dissemination, and communication of research widely to varied audiences, and to translate the findings into clinical practice (Grady & Gough, 2014, p. e26) with the goals of improving health outcomes. While many of the recommended key areas of research are mainly quantitative in nature, the use of qualitative methods and especially case study can help identify key variables and factors of self-care management that can

DOI: 10.4324/9781003435358-5

be tested. Since 2016, self-management of chronic conditions has been part of the NINR Strategic Plan.

Effective communication

"Drug overdose deaths have risen fivefold over the past two decades, and in 2021 106,699 deaths occurred. Between 2020 and 2021, the largest percentage increase in rates occurred among those aged 65 and over (28%)" (Spencer et al., 2022). The greatest barrier to substance-use disorder (SUD) screening, in large and small agencies is stigma (Zucker et al., 2018). Beginning in 2003, Substance Abuse and Mental Health Services Administration (SAMHSA) funded programs to roll out SUD education to medical and nursing professionals. This concept, screening, brief intervention, and referral to treatment (SBIRT) used motivational interviewing and change-talk to increase the effectiveness of the patient-provider interaction, thus increasing the likelihood of positive behavior change. These strategies impact self-care management.

Motivational interviewing

Motivational interviewing was developed in the early 1990s by Miller and Rollnick and takes a client-centered approach to therapy (2013). They emphasize that change is natural and that with therapeutic communication, persons struggling with behavior change can move toward resolving ambivalence. One strategy that is most helpful is using open-ended questions, affirming statements, reflecting both simple and complex, summarizing and informing and advising with permission (Miller & Rollnick, 2013, p. 72). The next steps in this process include using "change-talk" that creates an atmosphere in which a person can talk themselves into trying to change. Finally, providers help make a plan that works for the client. Doing something such as planning to reduce cigarette use by one per day is a positive start to changing behavior. Follow-up visits and possible referral to additional treatment, continue the relationship and commitment for change.

Transtheoretical model of change

Using Prochaska's stages of change model (Prochaska, et al., 1994), it is possible to engage with clients to create mutual trust, demonstrate respect and create an environment of change. The stages of change model include the stages labeled precontemplation, contemplation, preparation, action, and maintenance (p. 40). While not all persons move toward behavior change at the same rate, proceeding through these stages is necessary to maintain the desired change. While some people change for good, others may slip or lapse. The aim of using this model in conjunction with other self-care strategies is to help in assisting clients make difficult decisions about their health.

Nursing case studies and self-care management

As discussed in Chapter 4, improved health outcomes are the goal of care in health trajectory research. In the following section, self-care management studies that have examined health outcomes that were impacted by complex chronic conditions and in complex environments will be described. They illustrate challenges to self-care management of selected chronic conditions.

Case study and the vulnerability-stress model

The Biopsychosocial vulnerability-stress model illustrates the relationship of stress and vulnerability to health. Predisposition to illness coupled with impactful stressors may lead to illness and disability (Ingram & Luxton, 2005). Yin's (2009) multiple case study methodology offered the best approach in Maruca's (2016) case study research. Her research question was: "What are the similarities and differences of personal and environmental factors that contribute to psychological disorders and affect the health outcomes in the correctional population?" (p. 281). She applied the Biopsychosocial Vulnerability-Stress Model (Zubin & Spring, 1977) to better understand the impact of complex co-occurring conditions of incarcerated persons, on self-care behaviors and health outcomes.

In this study, the units of analysis were four "cases" of incarcerated persons with co-occurring diagnoses: (1) Anxiety and Substance Abuse, (2) Depression and Substance Abuse, (3) Antisocial and Substance Abuse, and (4) Bipolar and Substance Abuse (Maruca, 2016). Data were gathered from archival records at a securely identified correctional facility and approved by appropriate Institutional Review Boards. Using an extraction worksheet based on theory, data were collected and then transposed to an Excel format for analyses (see Table 5.1).

The data were then organized by pattern matching and using a cross-case thematic analysis (Yin, 2009). Emerging themes were (1) unstable, chaotic family life; (2) repeated incarcerations; and (3) ineffective coping skills. In three of four cases recidivism improved when the participant adhered to prescribed medications and treatment planning upon reentry. Trauma histories and disrupted family dynamics were also revealed. The within-case and across-case analyses supported the hypothesis that the greater personal vulnerabilities, less environmental stress is necessary for poor health outcomes. Individuals with co-occurring disease with incarceration experience and greater vulnerabilities fall into the category of poorer health outcomes. The results of this study demonstrated that the application of the Biopsychosocial Vulnerability-Stress Model to persons during and post-incarceration is beneficial as a research and clinical assessment tool, aiming to improve self-care behaviors and wellness.

Table 5.1 Case data extraction worksheet

Demographic	Age	Gender	Education	Marital status	Ethnicity	No data
Family history	Mental Illness	Substance Use	Violent Behavior	Types of Abuse	Source of Abuse	
Personal history	Mental Illness	Substance Use	Violent Behavior	Types of Abuse	Source of Abuse	
Medical history	Clinical visits	Medications	Treatment	Outcome		
Aggressive/Assaultive behavior	Age at occurrence	Prior to or during incarceration	Outcomes of Behavior (seclusion, charges pressed, etc.)	Treatment for behavior	No history of aggression or assault	
Number of disciplinary tickets	Reason	Risk score				
Criminal behavior	Offense	Severity of offense	Consequence	Escape history		
Employment history	Types of work	Length of employment	Disability benefits			
History of incarceration	Age at incarceration	Length of time incarcerated	Recidivism			
Social support	Number of visits during incarceration	Significance of social support (positive)	Family support (present, lacking)	Religious affiliation and support		
Housing	Type of housing	Homeless				
Discharge planning	Vocational needs	Follow-up treatment in place				

Case study and the biopsychosocial model

The goal of Lachance's case study (Lachance et al., 2023) was to gain an understanding of cannabis use among community-dwelling older adults. In addition to the psychoactive mind-altering property of use (e.g., getting high), there is limited information regarding older adults' perceptions of cannabis use in treating chronic conditions. Case study method was used to understand adult perceptions of cannabis use to treat chronic conditions such as insomnia, anxiety, and pain. The units of analysis were individuals who used cannabis, and the study findings were compared to findings from systematic reviews that studied the effectiveness of cannabis use for chronic conditions.

This study used the Biopsychosocial Model (BPSM) developed in the 1970s (Engel, 1981). The model places equal emphasis on the three dimensions of health and illness.

The theory proposes that a person's belief regarding illness is interconnected with their biological, psychological, and social environmental beliefs. The case study followed the four steps described by Siedlecki (2020). See Table 5.2.

Following the University IRB approval and informed verbal and written consent, data were collected through interviews with two older adults, using the BPSM theory as a guide in the interview process. "Once the interviews were completed, they were transcribed verbatim using *Otter.AI 2.3.113* translation software. The transcript was ingested into *Atlas.ti 9.1.3,* was coded using in vivo to identify categories and themes" (Lachance et al., 2003, p. 22). A critical aspect of a case study is searching for patterns in the data (Yin, 1981). Once the data was coded, a second level of coding was done mapping the information to the research questions and the BPSM. The following themes reflect the themes that emerged from the data: risks related to side effects (bio), lack of trust and autonomy (psycho), and prior use and cost (social).

Table 5.2 Case plan approach

1. Preparing and planning	2. Data Collection and data organization	3. Data analysis	4. Dissemination
○ Review the literature ○ Identify a theoretical framework ○ Identify the case(s) ○ Identify key information and informants	○ Interviews ○ Create a database	○ Analyze qualitative data ○ Look for triangulation ○ Identify themes	○ Organize findings

Patients felt that cannabis use was highly effective for treating their symptoms of chronic pain and insomnia, which is inconsistent with literature findings (Black et al., 2019; Longo et al., 2021; Suraev et al., 2020). The literature supports that patients should feel they have the right to make their own decisions (Davitt et al., 2016), in particular about prescribed medications (Kleinsinger, 2018). Compared to pharmaceutical pain medications and traditional therapies, both participants viewed cannabis products as less expensive, had fewer side effects, and gave them greater perceived autonomy over their health.

Nurses need to ensure that their patients are specifically asked about alternative therapies such as cannabis use is a preemptive step in successful self-care management. The goal for healthcare providers who work with older patients is to explore alternative therapies in addition to pharmaceutical medications. Providers are not trained to understand how much cannabis for a patient is too much. So even if they do disclose their use, further training is needed to guide the patient toward safe use.

Self-care management and the human-to-human relationship model

Prevention, early identification, and treatment options are needed to decrease the harm related to drug use. The nurse is often the first to interact with a person who injects drugs (PWID) in the healthcare setting. This interaction may influence the individual's disclosure of drug use, treatment engagement, and self-care management for future health-related issues. In 2015, Kim designed a case study strategy to describe the experience and the meaning attributed to the care of the PWID received by nurses in the acute care setting (Dion, 2019). Using Yin's (2014) case study approach, interviews were conducted with PWID from two diverse syringe access programs (SAPs) in economically, ethnically, and socially diverse areas. The unit of analysis for the study was any individual age 18 and older who spoke and understood English, had an encounter with a nurse on an inpatient medical unit, and was in active injection drug use. Following university and institutional review board approvals, open-ended semi-structured interview questions were used to guide the researcher in understanding the context and depth of each participant's story. The questions focused on the participant's experience with the received care, their interpretation of the meaning of this experience, and the impact the experience had or will have when they seek care the next time it is needed.

For this study, Joyce Travelbee's (1971) phases of the human-to-human relationship model served as in vivo codes. These phases include the original encounter, emerging identities, empathy, sympathy, ending in rapport building. Analyses occurred using participant checking during interviews and using a priori and in vivo codes. Transcripts were transcribed, deidentified, and listened to several times. *NVivo 10*, an electronic software used to collect and organize data, assisted with managing the data and categorizing themes.

The overarching themes were compared to the data several times throughout the analysis. Construct validity strategies included using two SAPs in geographically different areas, as this allowed for a sample of six different area hospitals. Additional construct validity strategies included audit reflexivity, member checking, using a content expert, and the contact summary form used after each interview. Internal validity strategies included pattern matching and addressing rival explanations. External validity strategies included triangulation and coding using Travelbee's (1971) phases of the development of rapport. Triangulation was performed by conducting the interviews at both SAPs to converge the data. Reliability strategies included using a case study protocol and case study database, a systematic archive of all the data from the case study (Yin, 2014). Data revealed several comparison cases and one rival case.

This systematic approach to analyzing the data allowed for understanding a complex real-life problem and the meaning of this experience for the PWID interviewed for this study. The theme of the rival case was *Understanding Addiction*. For the comparison cases, three themes and associated subthemes were discovered. The first theme of *Marginalization* and the subthemes of *Feelings of worthlessness*, *Mistrust*, and *Unpredictability of care* were examined. The second theme consisted of *Defensiveness*, the third theme of *Repeated Victimization*, and the subtheme of *Self-Care Management and Delay in Seeking Care*. Lastly, an outlier theme of *Young Enough to Be Saved* was explained.

Findings from this study supported that nurses needed more training to care for people with SUD. The participant who remained in the hospital the entire time stated they would not hesitate to seek care the next time it was needed. This contrasted with the comparison cases where most had left the hospital before receiving their fully prescribed treatment. In addition, the comparison cases either delayed seeking care or managed their care by seeking advice on the Internet rather than being subjected to the stigma they had experienced in the hospital.

Summary

Nurses must be sensitive to and trained in caring behaviors to develop a meaningful encounter with clients to facilitate self-care behaviors. In the previous examples, case study was used to uncover barriers to self-care management based on theoretical understandings. While several self-care instruments exist to measure this concept, case study methods are essential in outlining specific barriers to self-care. In addition, case study method emphasizes the need for up-to-date education, how to use motivational strategies and provide empathy and compassion, and to communicate more effectively. Respect is an essential behavior required by providers in caring for those with chronic health problems. The next chapter explores stigmatization and its relationship to self-care management.

References

Artiga, S., & Hinton, E. (2018). Beyond health care: The role of social determinants in promoting health and health equity. In *Issue Brief*. Henry J. Kaiser Family Foundation.

Black, N., Stockings, E., Campbell, G., Tran, L. T., Zagic, D., Hall, W. D., Farrell, M., & Degenhardt, L. (2019). Cannabinoids for the treatment of mental disorders and symptoms of mental disorders: A systematic review and meta-analysis. *The Lancet Psychiatry, 6*(12), 995–1010.

Corbin, J. M., & Strauss, A. (1985). Managing chronic illness at home: Three lines of work. *Qualitative Sociology, 8*(3), 224–247.

Corbin, J. M., & Strauss, A. (1991). A nursing model for chronic illness management based upon the trajectory framework. *Scholarly Inquiry for Nursing Practice, 5*(3), 155–174.

Davitt, J. K., Madigan, E. A., Rantz, M., & Skemp, L. (2016). Aging in community. *Research in Gerontological Nursing, 9*(1), 6–13. https://doi.org/10.3928/19404921-20151211-03

Dion, K. (2019). Perceptions of persons who inject drugs about nursing care they have received. *Journal of Addictions Nursing, 30*(2), 101–107. https://doi.org/10.1097/JAN.0000000000000277

Engel, G. L. (1981). The clinical application of the biopsychosocial model. *The Journal of Medicine and Philosophy, 6*, 101–123.

Fink, J. L., & Mercado, H. S. (2023). Health equity and accountability act of 2022 aims to combat disparities. *Pharmacy Times, 89*(5). https://www.pharmacytimes.com/view/health-equity-and-accountability-act-of-2022-aims-to-combat-disparities

Grady, P. A., & Gough, L. L. (2014). Self-management: A comprehensive approach to management of chronic conditions. *American Journal of Public Health, 104*(8), e25–e31.

Iezzoni, L. I. (2010). Multiple chronic conditions and disabilities: Implications for health services research and data demands. *Health Services Research, 45*(5 Pt 2), 1523–1540. https://doi.org/10.1111/j.1475-6773.2010.01145.x

Ingram, R. E., & Luxton, D. D. (2005). Vulnerability-stress models. In B. L. Hankin & J. R. Z. Abela (Eds.), *Development of psychopathology. A vulnerability-stress perspective*. Sage Publications.

Kleinsinger, F. (2018). The unmet challenge of medication nonadherence. *Permanente Journal, 22*(3), 83–85. https://doi.org/10.7812/TPP/18-033

Lachance, S. L., Zucker, D. M., & Hutchins, J. M. (2023). Adult cannabis use: An exploratory case study. *Journal of Gerontological Nursing, 49*(8), 19–26. https://doi.org/10.3928/00989134-20230707-01

Longo, R., Oudshoorn, A., & Befus, D. (2021). Cannabis for chronic pain: A rapid systematic review of randomized control trials. *Pain Management Nursing, 22*(2), 141–149.

Maruca, A. T. (2016). A case study using the biopsychosocial vulnerability-stress model as a framework to understand the incarceration experience. *Journal for Evidence-Based Practice in Correctional Health, 1*(1), 276–312.

Miller, W. R., & Rollnick, S. (2013). *Motivational interviewing: Helping people change* (3rd ed.). Guilford Press.

Orem, D. E. (2001). *Nursing concepts of practice* (6th ed.). Mosby.

Prochaska, J. O., Velicer, W. F., Rossi, J. S., Goldstein, M. G., Marcus, B. H., Rakowski, W., Fiore, C. Harlow, L. L., Redding, C. A., Rosenbloom, D., & Rossi, S. R. (1994). Stages of change and decisional balance for 12 problem behaviors. *Health Psychology*, *13*(1), 39–46.

Siedlecki, S. L. (2020). Case study research design in nursing. *Clinical Nurse Specialist, 34*(6), 250–256.

Spencer, M. R., Miniño, A. M., & Warner, M. (2022). Drug overdose deaths in the United States, 2001–2021. In *NCHS data brief, no 457*. National Center for Health Statistics. https://doi.org/10.15620/cdc:122556

Suraev, A. S., Marshall, N. S., Vandrey, R., McCartney, D., Benson, M. J., McGregor, I. S., Grunstein, R. R., & Hoyos, C. M. (2020). Cannabinoid therapies in the management of sleep disorders: A systematic review of pre-clinical and clinical studies. *Sleep Medicine Reviews*, *53*, 101339. https://doi.org/10.1016/j.smrv.2020.101339

Travelbee, J. (1971). *Interpersonal aspects of nursing* (2nd ed.). F.A. Davis.

Yin, R. K. (1981). The case study as a serious research strategy. *Science Communication*, *3*(1), 97–114. https://doi.org/10.1177/107554708100300106

Yin, R. K. (2009). *Case study research: Design and methods* (4th ed.). Sage Publications.

Yin, R. K. (2014). *Case study research design and methods* (5th ed.). Sage Publications.

Zubin, J., & Spring, B. (1977). Vulnerability: A new view of schizophrenia. *Journal of Abnormal Psychology, 86*(2), 103–126. https://doi.org/10.1037/0021-843X.86.2.103

Zucker, D. M., Chandler, G. E., Rataj, S., Dundon, E., Heffernan, D., DiFulvio, G., Fedorchak, D., & Linowski, S. (2018). Uncovering stigma. SBIRT promotes whole curriculum learning. *Journal of Addictions Nursing, Letter to the Editor*, *29*(3), 203–204.

6 Stigmatization

Donna M. Zucker

Background and anti-stigma models

The National Alliance on Mental Health (NAMI) (n.d.) describes the origins of stigma and defines it as holding a person responsible for a symptom or condition, who is fraught with uncertainty or unpredictability, and may be dangerous and incompetent. In order to assist persons with stigmatizing chronic conditions such as mental illness, eliminating labels, stereotyping, and prejudice within the communities we serve must be a priority. Only then can we achieve health equity. Attention to civil rights and health disparities have drawn attention to stigma, and several models exist aimed at ameliorating stigma. The following are evidence-based examples that may be useful to nurses and healthcare providers in a wide variety of settings.

Framework integrating normative influences on stigma (FINIS)

Pescosolido et al. (2008) believe that stigma is central to community and individual characteristics, particularly when answers to illness and other social problems are needed. They developed the FINIS to illustrate and describe this combination of factors. They offer strategies to positively impact stigmatizing illnesses, such as mental illness and substance-use disorder, among others. Stigma is shaped through a variety of factors and experiences. Among the anti-stigma models, the one created by Pescosolido et al. (2008) described a structure that considers a variety of influences on stigma. It is comprised of the individual factors or micro level, the treatment system or meso-level and the community or macro level.

The micro level of stigma includes public stigma such as stereotyping, prejudice, and discrimination toward others, as well as self-stigma or negative self-belief, low-esteem, and negative behavioral responses to prejudice. The meso-level stigmatization impacts treatment. Examples of these impacts can be negative (labeling) or positive (adoption of institutional policies and structures to address cultures of stigma). The macro level includes societal impacts of stigmatization and are also either positive (using first-person language, building social networks and integration) or negative (adopting stigmatizing ideologies

DOI: 10.4324/9781003435358-6

that send negative messages and values about a group or groups in the community). There are multiple ways to curb, and halt continued stereotypes through community education, role-play, and institutional policies and procedures.

Pescosolido and Martin (2015) point out the need for more accurate measurement and conceptual definitions of stigma. The FINIS model aims to distill the essential concepts of stigma into three broad categories in hopes of improving measurement and interventions. Model authors state that compared to the individual and the community levels, the literature has focused little attention on the healthcare system's impact on stigma. This model is a systems science approach considering individual and societal systems that are dynamic in nature.

Understanding stigmatizing influences is aimed at reducing poor health outcomes. While elaborate and multifaceted, the FINIS can assist clinicians and educators in several ways: to first and foremost emphasize that stigma is an ever-present component of care giving; to provide competency training; and to provide an evidence-based model for ongoing research and testing. It is unlikely that stigma will be eliminated but for those with chronic illness, such a model may provide healthcare providers with strategies to help them maintain a healthy life.

Motivation and Opportunity and DEterminants (MODE) model

Nearly two decades ago Fazio (1990) developed the MODE model. It was seen as a guiding framework for the many processes by which behaviors are guided by attitude. This is a dual process model, which means that it offers two paths, one focused on deliberate processes and the other on spontaneous processes. The model proposes that under the correct circumstances (opportunity and motivation) that behavior will be predicated by a deliberate attitudinal process. If one or the other of these circumstances is missing, then the behavior will be predicted spontaneously.

As an example, according to Olson and Fazio, "Individuals low in motivation to control racial prejudice, individuals with more pro-White attitudes, automatically activated racial attitudes and rated White (relative to Black) targets more favorably." Individuals with more pro-Black attitudes automatically activated racial attitudes toward Black targets (Zabel & Seacat, 2021, pp. 258–259). This model has been in use for over 20 years and has been included as a chapter in many texts of dual process theories. The model has been applied in a variety of contexts including health decision-making (Ajzen & Fishbein, 2005).

Process model for designing and delivering successful anti-stigma programs for healthcare providers

A grounded theory model for reducing stigma in Canadian health professionals was developed as part of a national initiative titled, *Opening Minds*

(Knaak & Patten, 2016). One aim of the program was to "help reduce the stigma of mental illness" (p. 54) by developing anti-stigma programs for healthcare providers. The study included results of 23 in-depth interviews, follow-up individual interviews, review of documents and direct observation. Using a grounded theory approach, a model emerged. The model is composed of four processes: set up for success, build the program using key ingredients, make the connection, and work toward culture change targeting the roots of healthcare provider stigma and offering tools for success through interactive education. System level change is acknowledged as a key point of emphasis, yet addressing individual stigma and held biases were the focus of this framework for change.

In a data synthesis of evaluation studies (Knaak et al., 2014) it was found that six components had to be present for optimal program effectiveness. They are (1) that the program should include social contact in the form of a personal testimony of a speaker with the lived experience of mental illness, (2) that the program should employ multiple forms or points of social contact (for example, a presentation from a live speaker and a video presentation), multiple first-voice speakers, multiple points of social contact between program participants and people with lived experience of mental illness, (3) that the program should focus on behavior change by teaching skills that help healthcare providers know what to say and what to do, (4) that the program should engage in myth-busting, (5) that the program should use an enthusiastic facilitator or instructor who models a person-centered approach (that is a person-first perspective as opposed to a pathology-first perspective) to set the tone and guide program messaging, and (6) that the program should emphasize and demonstrate recovery as a key part of its messaging (pS22).

An assessment and intervention model of health-related stigma

This model was based on the early work of Weiss who studied the stigma related to disfiguring neglected tropical skin diseases, such as leprosy (2008). His foundational work in this area was based on the work of Scambler (1998). Scambler posited that the model "hinges on a distinction between enacted and felt stigma. Enacted stigma refers to actual discrimination or unacceptability, whereas felt stigma refers to the fear of such discrimination" (p. 1054). Weiss extended that thinking "by differentiating *anticipated* stigma (regarded as unjustified but likely) and *internalized* stigma." In this sense, "internalization refers to a process in which a person with a stigmatized condition accepts perceived exclusionary views of society and self-stigmatizes himself or herself" (p. e237). The goals of this work are to suggest further study and interventions for people both stigmatized by health conditions, and the community at large, including those in positions to impact health policy. The authors are proponents of using generic stigma instruments whenever possible.

In 2019, this model was expanded yet again (van Brakel et al., 2019) to emphasize those who are stigmatized and those who are the source of the stigma. This modified model includes the addition of specific interventions. The language and ideas are more generic and suggest that regardless of measurement tool, the interventions have overall been successfully used to measure or address stigma across a variety of conditions. For example, for people who are stigmatized it is suggested that counseling, skills building, and empowerment are important interventions. For the sources of stigma, such as the community, healthcare staff, structures, policies and laws, the model encourages education, contact with the affected person(s), and work with change agents and popular opinion leaders (van Brakel et al., 2019, p. 3).

Summary

While these four examples do not represent the entirety of anti-stigma models, they represent promise for nursing care of persons with chronic conditions. Frameworks and models such as these create a blueprint for the provider and client. These models also focus on attitudes and behavior. Additionally, attention is focused on the individual (stigmatized and stigmatizer) as the recipient of education or assistance. Finally, while structural and societal changes are key, they seem less attended to in the literature than attention to the individual. Of note, the model by Knaak and Patten outlines essential characteristics of providing anti-stigma education to promote relationship, trust, and empathy. The model by van Brakel includes key interventions for both those who are stigmatized and the sources of stigma. In total any of these models can influence the case study researcher, as they engage with the client, community, or organization, remembering that sensitivity to stigma is a first step in relationship building.

References

Ajzen, I., & Fishbein, M. (2005). The influence of attitudes on behavior. In D. Albarracin, B. T. Johnson, & M. O. Zanna (Eds.), *The handbook of attitudes* (pp. 173–221). Lawrence Erlbaum Associates.

Clair, M. (2018). Stigma. In J. M. Ryan (Ed.), *Core concepts in sociology* (pp. 318–321). Wiley Blackwell.

Corrigan, P. W., & Watson, A. C. (2002). Understanding the impact of stigma on people with mental illness. *World Psychiatry*, *1*(1), 16–20.

Fazio, R. H. (1990). Multiple processes by which attitudes guide behavior: The MODE model as an integrative framework. In M. P. Zanna (Ed.), *Advances in experimental social psychology* (Vol. 23, pp. 75–109). Academic Press.

Goffman, E. (1963). *Stigma: Notes on the management of spoiled identity*. Simon & Schuster.

Knaak, S., Modgill, G., & Patten, S. B. (2014). Key ingredients of anti-stigma programs for health care providers: A data synthesis of evaluative studies. *The Canadian Journal of Psychiatry*, *59*(suppl 1), 19–26. https://doi.org/10.1177/070674371405901S06

Knaak, S., & Patten, S. (2016). A grounded theory model for reducing stigma in health professionals in Canada. *Acta Psychiatrica Scandinavica*, *134*(suppl 446), 53–62.

NAMI. (n.d.). *Stigma free*. National Alliance on Mental Illness. Retrieved September 27, 2023, from https://nami.org/Get-Involved/Pledge-to-Be-StigmaFree?gad=1

Olson, M. A., & Fazio, R. H. (2004). Trait inferences as a function of automatically activated racial attitudes and motivation to control prejudiced reactions. *Basic and Applied Social Psychology*, *26*(1), 1–11. https://doi.org/10.1207/s15324834basp2601_1

Parcesepe, A. M., & Cabassa, L. J. (2013). Public stigma of mental illness in the United States: A systematic literature review. *Administration and Policy in Mental Health and Mental Health Services Research*, *40*(5). https://doi.org/10.1007/s10488-012-0430-z

Pescosolido, B. A., & Martin, J. K. (2015). The stigma complex. *Annual Review of Sociology*, *41*, 87–116.

Pescosolido, B. A., Martin, J. K., Lang, A., & Olafsdottir, S. (2008). Rethinking theoretical approaches to stigma: A framework integrating normative influences on stigma (FINIS). *Social Science and Medicine*, *67*, 431–440.

Quinn, D., & Earnshaw, V. (2011). Understanding concealable stigmatized identities: The role of identity in psychological, physical, and behavioral outcomes. *Social Issues and Policy Review*, *5*(1), 160–190.

Quinn, D., & Earnshaw, V. (2013). Concealable stigmatized identities and psychological well-being. *Social and Personality Psychology Compass*, *7*, 40–51. https://doi.org/10.1111/spc3.12005

Scambler, G. (1998). Stigma and disease: Changing paradigms. *The Lancet*, *352*(9133), 1054–1055.

van Brakel, W. H., Cataldo, J., Grover, S., Kohrt, B. A., Nyblade, L., Stockton, M., Wouters, E., & Yang, L. H. (2019). Out of the silos: Identifying cross-cutting features of health-related stigma to advance measurement and intervention. *BMC Medicine*, *17*(13), 1–17.

Weiss, M. G. (2008). Stigma and the social burden of neglected tropical diseases. *PLoS Neglected Tropical Disease*, *2*(5), e237. https://doi.org/10.1371/journal.pntd.0000237; https://journals.plos.org/plosntds/article?id=10.1371/journal.pntd.0000237

Zabel, K. L. & Seacat, J. D. (2021). Self-protection and correction for automatically activated weight-bias: Revisiting the applicability of the MODE model. *Journal of Applied Social Psychology*, *53*, 257–269.

7 Application to clinical problem solving

Donna M. Zucker, Annette Maruca,
Sonya LaChance, and Kimberly Dion

Stigma and self-care exemplars

Adult cannabis use

In the case study conducted with older adults who use cannabis (Lachance et al., 2023), two participants demonstrated a high degree of self-care initiative in choosing and using cannabis to alleviate pain and insomnia. Both participants conveyed their perception that pharmaceutical companies were not the only solution to treating chronic health conditions. They perceived that cannabis was "more natural and that they had more control over the dosage." One participant felt that the relationship between the medical community and pharmaceutical companies was not about health but drug industry profits. With cannabis use, participants got to the point of figuring out the right products and the right amount for managing their condition. Their sense of autonomy and control were latent themes contributing to the use of cannabis. For both participants self-management of pain was related to their control of the dose. These findings are inconsistent with systematic reviews on cannabis use by patients with anxiety, pain, and insomnia (Black et al., 2019; Longo et al., 2021; Suraev et al., 2020). Despite the lack of evidence that cannabis relieves chronic pain, patients' perception of benefit outweighs the harm (Longo et al., 2021).

As discussed in Chapter 4, attention to the patient's perceived versus actual functional status is an important component of the patient-provider relationship. Healthcare providers need to remain open-minded when discussing issues with their patients. Recognizing that adverse reactions to pharmaceutical medications impact a patient's quality of life should also be considered and taken seriously when a patient raises it as a concern. Side effects often contribute to the feelings, thoughts, and behaviors that drive the patient toward alternative therapies. Other recommended strategies include ensuring that the patient is specifically asked about alternative therapies such as cannabis, as a preemptive step. The goal for healthcare providers should

DOI: 10.4324/9781003435358-7

be to work with older patients to explore alternative therapies in addition to pharmaceutical medications. It also allows the provider to help identify and discuss potential health problems and adverse side effects. Patients must be regularly screened for cannabis use in primary care (Bertram et al., 2020) providing an opportunity for education and reinforcing safety.

Co-morbid conditions while incarcerated

In Maruca's (2016) case study, she explored the association between co-occurring diagnoses, antisocial traits, and challenging behaviors within the incarcerated population. In a review by Sarteschi (2013), it was determined that half or more of all persons with an incarceration experience had problems with their mental health. Maruca's study described cases with four co-occurring mental health conditions: anxiety and substance abuse, depression and substance abuse, antisocial and substance abuse, and bipolar and substance abuse. For those persons with antisocial and substance-use disorders, there were prevalent behavioral patterns of "use of alcohol or substances starting at a young age, exaggerated emotional dysregulation and or aggression/violence" (p. 295). Seeking and refusing treatment were noted in several instances, often resulting in worsening symptoms. During their incarceration, treatment plans were in place and those individuals who adhered to them had better health outcomes. Structured programs offered upon release saw similar results. Finally, individuals with established discharge healthcare plans and social support systems fared better upon re-entering the community.

Perceptions of persons who inject drugs care while hospitalized

The literature has described how people who inject drugs (PWID) are stigmatized within our communities. It is common that PWID do not differentiate care delivered by a doctor, nurse, or pharmacist and group healthcare professionals (HCPs) together. Nurses, however, spend the most hours per day with PWID when hospitalized. In Dion's 2015 case study of PWIDs' perceptions of received care, HCPs were reported to have given less than average care to PWIDs (Dion, 2019). Strong biases and prejudice against PWID result in their mistrust of HCP. In a study by McCreaddie et al. (2010), HCP behaviors toward PWID included breach of confidentiality and speaking down in a derogatory manner. However, not all HCPs were described as "bad," and some were rated as "good." In Dion's study it was noted that received care at a syringe access program was very different from hospital care as participants were met with nonjudgmental and nonstigmatizing care. Study participants made comments about expecting a poor reception when seeking medical care often leading to delaying treatment.

All the participants described how they attempted to self-manage their healthcare needs, or just ignored their health, to avoid having to seek care from an HCP. Their experiences receiving healthcare were described as overall negative. Repeated cycles of trauma negatively impacted their wellness trajectory. Several of the participants described the effects of these interactions as the reason for their increased depression, feelings of worthlessness, increased drug usage, and avoidance of seeking healthcare when it was needed. Recommended interventions are to ensure that providers are educated in addiction and how to care for persons with this chronic condition. Support, empathy, and compassion are essential to create a therapeutic environment of care. Additionally, a culture change in the institution is necessary to set the tone for equitable healthcare delivery.

Conclusion

The case studies highlighted in this book have demonstrated the day-to-day experiences of persons with a wide range of chronic health problems. In all cases stigma negatively impacted their self-care efforts and health. Stigma is pervasive in our society. The literature has emphasized that one's attitude and behavior can lead to both negative and positive actions and under the right conditions can become normalized. Efforts to act as a change agent in our work and social settings is an imperative in healthcare settings. The consequence for our patients results in better health outcomes. Anti-stigma models must be in place to provide information, education, and possible interventions that include caring and nonjudgmental approaches to creating relationships with clients. Stigmatized patients need to feel unafraid and unashamed to seek care. They need empathy, a caring reception, resources, and structured support systems. Change can occur at the individual, system, and community levels with education and administrative support to enact a culture change.

Despite the differences in various chronic conditions, whether they be aging, mental illness or addiction, barriers to self-care were evident and were often accompanied by stigmatization. Anti-stigma models are useful for planning care with clients, by developing interventions that work with the client where they are in their health trajectory. Table 7.1 illustrates key themes from the three case studies discussed, wherein self-care and stigma were overlapping concepts. Anti-stigma model elements and strategies to improve health outcomes are offered.

Table 7.1 Case studies in which stigma and self-care coexist, anti-stigma model elements and strategies to improve outcomes

Author	Population	Stigma	Self-care	FINIS level	MODE model	Process model	Assessment and intervention model	Summary suggested strategies
Dion (2019)	Persons who inject drugs	Communication, behaviors, and treatment from healthcare providers	No medical education; rely on friends and internet.	–Individual – public and self-stigma. –Treatment System.	–Healthcare providers with negative attitudes about addiction have stigmatizing behaviors	–Educate resources and using person-first and those with lived experience	–Experienced stigma and enacted stigma. –Information and education needed	–Provider education –Administrative culture change
Maruca (2016)	Incarcerated and mentally ill	Repeated incarceration and co-existing poor mental health	Disrupted re-integration into the community after incarceration	–Community and Treatment System	–Employers, landlords, and healthcare clinics with negative attitudes about incarceration have stigmatizing behaviors	–Educate community programs should employ multiple forms or points of social contact	–Experienced stigma. –Information required for resource persons/ change agents in the community. –Client skill building, and empowerment	Community messaging Policies to enable access resources
Lachance et al. (2023)	Persons who use cannabis for chronic pain	Lack of trust in the pharmaceutical industry	Do their own research and trial and error in finding the appropriate dose	–Treatment system –Community	–Opportunity and highly motivated to take on self-care behaviors	Educate providers with skills in communicating and taking informed action	–Anticipated stigma –Negative attitudes and polices and –Laws and polices a source of stigma	Provider education: accurate facts about cannabis to stay safe

References

Bertram, J. R., Porath, A., Seitz, D., Kalant, H., Krishnamoorthy, A., Nickerson, J., Sidhu, A., Smith, A., & Teed, R. (2020). Canadian guidelines on cannabis use disorder among older adults. *Canadian Geriatrics Journal*, *23*(1), 135–142. https://doi.org/10.5770/cgj.23.424

Black, N., Stockings, E., Campbell, G., Tran, L. T., Zagic, D., Hall, W. D., Farrell, M., & Degenhardt, L. (2019). Cannabinoids for the treatment of mental disorders and symptoms of mental disorders: A systematic review and meta-analysis. *The Lancet Psychiatry*, *6*(12), 995–1010.

Creswell, J. (1998). *Qualitative inquiry and research design. Choosing among five traditions.* Sage Publications.

Dion, K. (2019). Perceptions of persons who inject drugs about nursing care they have received. *Journal of Addictions Nursing*, *30*(2), 101–107. https://doi.org/10.1097/JAN.0000000000000277

Lachance, S. L., Zucker, D. M., & Hutchins, J. M. (2023). Adult cannabis use: An exploratory case study. *Journal of Gerontological Nursing*, *49*(8), 19–26. https://doi.org/10.3928/00989134-20230707-01

Longo, R., Oudshoorn, A., & Befus, D. (2021). Cannabis for chronic pain: A rapid systematic review of randomized control trials. *Pain Management Nursing*, *22*(2), 141–149.

Maruca, A. T. (2016). A case study using the biopsychosocial vulnerability-stress model as a framework to understand the incarceration experience. *Journal for Evidence-Based Practice in Correctional Health*, *1*(1), 276–312.

McCreaddie, M., Lyons, I., Watt, D., Ewing, E., Croft, J., Smith, M., & Tocher, J. (2010). Routines and rituals: A grounded theory of the pain management of drug users in acute care settings. *Journal of Clinical Nursing*, *19*(19–20), 2730–2740. https://doi.org/10.1111/j.1365-2702.2010.03284.x

Sarteschi, C. M. (2013, July–September). Mentally ill offenders involved with the U.S. criminal justice system: A synthesis. *Sage Open*, 1–11. https://doi.org/10.1177/2158244013497029

Suraev, A. S., Marshall, N. S., Vandrey, R., McCartney, D., Benson, M. J., McGregor, I. S., Grunstein, R. R., & Hoyos, C. M. (2020). Cannabinoid therapies in the management of sleep disorders: A systematic review of preclinical and clinical studies. *Sleep Medicine Reviews*, *53*.

Yin, R. K. (2014). *Case study research design and methods* (5th ed.). Sage Publications.

8 Current and future nursing directions

Donna M. Zucker

Appreciative inquiry

Appreciative inquiry (AI) reframes the question, "What is wrong and how do we fix it?" to "What are we best at and let's have more of that!" (May et al., 2021, p. 464). Several experts in AI have demonstrated success in training industry employees in this approach to culture change and to improve the workplace (Adams et al., 2007; Cooperrider & Whitney, 1999; Hammond, 2013; Whitney & Trosten-Bloom, 2003). The AI process can be short or long with groups or individuals and each iteration will be unique. Once all members of the community or organization are engaged in the process and begins with setting the affirmative topics. Four essential phases of the process are discovery, dream, design, and destiny. The discovery phase mobilizes all the stakeholders in articulating the strengths and best practices. The dreaming phase creates the opportunity to envision the future. The design phase allows for propositions of what the ideal organization could be like. During the final phase, destiny, the participants encourage hope for ongoing positive change, as well as sustaining a high level of performance (Cooperrider & Whitney, 2005, pp. 62–65). It is my belief that using AI and case method in combination will transform the action research landscape in examining chronic health issues, particularly in the most vulnerable.

AI and current nursing care

Among the health disparities discussed in this book, the management of chronic illness issues is very challenging for clients and providers. The literature was explored to determine how AI is used in nursing care and healthcare, and what outcomes can be translated into nursing clinical practice from an AI innovation. A search of databases CINAHL, PyschInfo, Social Sciences Abstracts, and PubMed was limited to peer-reviewed journals and doctoral dissertations for years 2013–2023. References were scanned for additional articles. Keywords AI AND patient care and AI AND nursing care resulted in six titles that met inclusion criteria. Upon reading the full texts, one was a

DOI: 10.4324/9781003435358-8

review of literature, and three studies alluded to using "discovering and appreciating," the first step of the 4-D cycle process but did not refer to the model thereafter (Affleck et al., 2022; Morgan et al., 2017; Wilson et al., 2023). Two papers described using AI Innovation accurately and completely (Falk, 2013; Havers et al., 2006). Using an action research approach, Falk examined "the existing strength and effectiveness in a nurse-mentoring program for children with incarcerated parents" (p. 7). In using all four steps of the 4-D process the author developed, across two years, a nurse-mentoring program model curriculum. Havers and colleagues took a similar research approach to "create a service-research partnership with six community hospitals. The project goal is to build capacity to use what research tells us to shape practice environments to enhance nurse retention and quality patient care" (p. 463). Across five years, the authors overcame initial challenges and organizational change took place in nursing and other departments that adopted the AI process. Impacts were on improved workplace structures as well as positive communication.

Examples of AI healthcare

An integrative review of using AI of inpatient nursing settings revealed that eight studies met inclusion criteria as integrating the 4-D cycle (Watkins et al., 2017). They discovered only one study in eight, achieved transformation by including an appreciated inquiry intervention into diverse units in an acute care setting. The interventions included "being courageous, connecting emotionally, being curious, collaborating, considering other perspectives, compromising and celebrating" (p. 184).

May et al. (2021) utilized this model to create a change throughout several departments within the University of Virginia Health Sciences System. In healthcare the dynamic and fluid environment has created job dissatisfaction among nursing and medical students. May and colleagues outlined two strategies of AI and practice to address two system-wide issues, discriminatory behavior, and burnout. As an outcome of embedding AI processes into their system, they created two positive programs. One is a program to foster healthy teams, focused on self-care and reducing stressors. The second is a series of videos and online trainings to combat workplace bias and discrimination.

Concluding remarks

The need for understanding and examination of human phenomenon not easily measured requires research methods that incorporate an emphasis on health equity and compassion. Persons with chronic health problems may or may not have access to healthcare. They also can suffer disparities that decrease health access and a good quality of life. Of significance is that six in ten Americans live with at least one chronic condition (CDC, 2023), and the World Health

Organization reports that non-communicable diseases claim approximately 3/4 or all lives lost each year (UN News, 2023).

Case study method has been seen as a viable, emerging, and rigorous research method. It is especially useful within the nursing context for examining the experiences of the voiceless, the stigmatized and those experiencing health disparities. Commonalities across these chapters are the evolution of case method as an important research method, especially when junior researchers are given the proper mentoring and education. Future case study research must examine human phenomena through a health equity lens. One appropriate adjunct is the use of AI in examining the affirmative topic, appreciating what is working well, what is envisioned for the future, make a decision to get there and maintain the excitement to sustain the change. Current case study outcomes in this book include harm reduction, recovery-oriented and trauma-informed care. These are strength-based interventions that promote autonomy, self-care, and wellness trajectories. The inclusion of AI processes can only help individuals achieve wellness.

References

Adams, W. A., Cady, S., Devane, T., & Holman, P. (2007). *The change handbook: The definitive resource on today's best methods for engaging whole systems*. Berrett-Koehler Publishers.

Affleck, F., Hung, L., & Phinney, A. (2022). Reaching out to those we teach about: A qualitative appreciative inquiry of older persons' experience as mentors in a bachelor of nursing programme during the Covid-19 pandemic. *International Practice Development Journal*, *12*(2). https://www.fons.org/library/journal-ipdj-home

CDC. (n.d.). *Chronic disease*. National Center for Chronic Disease Prevention and Health Promotion. Retrieved May 8, 2023, from https://www.cdc.gov/chronicdisease/

Cooperrider, D. L., & Whitney, D. (1999). *Appreciative inquiry: Collaborating for change*. Berrett-Koehler.

Cooperrider, D. L., & Whitney, D. (2005). *Appreciative inquiry. A positive revolution in change*. Berrett-Koehler.

Falk, K. (2013). *Appreciative inquiry to transform nursing practice for mentoring children of promise* [Dissertation]. ProQuest. UMI Number: 3561585.

Hammond, S. A. (2013). *The thin book of appreciative inquiry* (3rd ed.). The Thin Book Publishing Co. ISBN: 0-9665373-1-9

Havers, D. S., Wood, S. O., & Leeman, J. (2006). Improving nursing practice and patient care. Building capacity with appreciative inquiry. *Journal of Nursing Administration, 36*(10), 463–470.

May, N. B., Haizlip, J., & Plews-Ogan, M. (2021). Changing the conversation: Appreciative inquiry and appreciative practices in healthcare. In S. McNamee, M. Gergen, C. Camargo-Borges, & E. Rasera (Eds.), *The SAGE handbook of social constructionist practice* (pp. 464–475). Sage Publications.

Morgan, S. J., Pullon, S. R., MacDonald, L. M., McKinlay, E. M., & Gray, B. V. (2017). Case study observational research: A framework for conducting case study research where observational data are the focus. *Qualitative Health Research, 27*(7), 1060–1068.

UN News. (2023). *Chronic diseases taking 'immense and increasing toll on lives', warns WHO.* United Nations. https://news.un.org/en/story/2023/05/1136832

Watkins, S., Dewar, B., & Kennedy, C. (2017). Appreciative inquiry as an intervention to change nursing practice in in-patient settings: An integrative review. *International Journal of Nursing Studies, 60,* 179–190.

Whitney, D. K. & Trosten-Bloom, A. (2003). *The Power of Appreciative Inquiry.* San Francisco, CA: Berrett-Koehler Publishing, Inc.

Wilson, B., Crandall, J., & Harwood, L. (2023). Successful home hemodialysis programs: An exploration of key nursing care processes. *Nephrology Nursing Journal, 50*(3), 215–224.

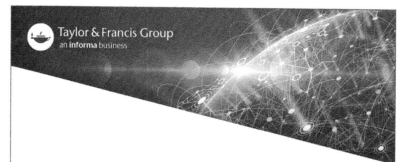

For Product Safety Concerns and Information please contact our EU representative GPSR@taylorandfrancis.com Taylor & Francis Verlag GmbH, Kaufingerstraße 24, 80331 München, Germany

Printed and bound by CPI Group (UK) Ltd, Croydon, CR0 4YY
01/05/2025
01858503-0001